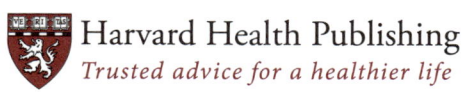

Dear Reader,

If you've ever twisted your knee, cut your finger, or been stung by an insect, you have personal experience with inflammation. The familiar sensations of pain, redness, swelling, and heat that result from an injury or infection are hallmarks of the inflammatory process. Inflammation represents an essential survival mechanism that helps the body fight off hostile microbes and repair tissues damaged in injuries. Yet there is another side of inflammation that can be harmful rather than helpful to human health. There's evidence that inflammation is involved in a number of disease processes.

As a rheumatologist at Beth Israel Deaconess Medical Center, I have seen the harmful side of inflammation in my patients firsthand. It can cause joint swelling, pain, and reduced mobility. The trigger for such inflammation is often an autoimmune disease, such as rheumatoid arthritis or psoriatic arthritis. Today, we are fortunate to have numerous weapons against autoimmune-induced inflammation in our treatment arsenal—drugs that not only relieve symptoms, but actually halt the disease process, even if they don't cure it.

Less obvious inflammation also simmers beneath the surface in millions of other Americans. This low-grade inflammation—which is fueled by both genetic influences and lifestyle factors like a poor diet, a lack of exercise, and excess weight—contributes to many of the most insidious and deadly diseases we face today—among them heart disease, cancer, Alzheimer's disease, and other forms of dementia. In cases like these, the same inflammatory response that was designed to protect us against infectious agents like bacteria and viruses turns against us.

This report is designed to be your guide to the most common causes of inflammation and the many conditions that trigger it. In the following pages, you'll learn the signs of conditions that are obviously linked to inflammation, from autoimmune diseases such as inflammatory bowel disease and rheumatoid arthritis, to common problems that people often don't realize have an inflammatory component, such as heart disease and dementia. More importantly, you'll gain an understanding of the types of interventions that most effectively combat them, and you will learn highly effective, evidence-based strategies you can implement every day to dampen inflammation before it can lead to disease.

Sincerely,

Robert H. Shmerling, M.D.
Medical Editor

Inflammation: Friend or foe (or both)?

The more scientists learn about the human body, the more extraordinary it seems. Composed of some 37 trillion cells, it performs a multitude of tasks with astonishing strength and precision. The examples are innumerable. The eyes can distinguish 10 million colors. The thighbone can withstand 6,000 pounds of compressive force. The heart has the power to pump 2,000 gallons of blood each day, sometimes against the pull of gravity—and it does so day in and day out, decade after decade.

The body also comes equipped with a built-in defense system—a complex army of infection-fighting cells and proteins that warn other cells of invaders, fight them off when they arrive, and heal any damage the resulting conflict produces. Inflammation is an important part of this defensive system and one that is essential for our survival.

You've seen the effects of inflammation in real time if you've ever gotten a paper cut, sprained your ankle, or been stung by a bee. The word comes from the Latin verb *inflammare*, which means "to set on fire." The name is fitting, given that redness and heat are two of the signs that an ancient Roman physician noted in the first century, when he became the first person to document this phenomenon (see "A brief history of inflammation," page 3). The redness and heat, along with pain and swelling that result from an injury or infection, are evidence of the inflammatory process under way beneath the skin's surface. Not visible but similar in process is the inflammation that results when you come down with an infection like the flu or pneumonia. In both cases, the immune system is waging a battle inside your body against invading microbes. Without its defenses, a minor cut or illness could quickly turn deadly.

However, the powerful weapon of inflammation is not always directed at outside invaders. Sometimes the immune system misfires and turns against the body itself, launching an autoimmune response that manifests in diseases like lupus, rheumatoid arthritis, psoriasis, and multiple sclerosis. These problems are dramatic and quite obvious. In type 1 diabetes, for example, the immune system attacks specialized cells in the pancreas, crippling the body's ability to produce the hormone insulin.

Fortunately, the proportion of the population affected by autoimmune diseases is relatively small. But almost everyone is potentially affected by a much broader range of inflammatory problems. A growing body of evidence suggests that low-grade, chronic inflammation—the kind that can simmer for decades

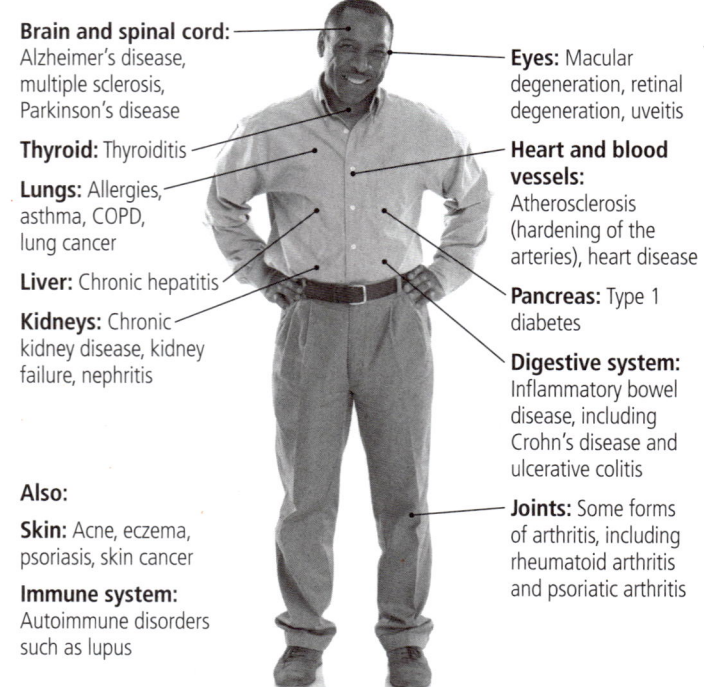

Figure 1: Diseases linked to chronic inflammation

When you have chronic inflammation, your body is in a constant state of high alert. The release of inflammatory chemicals can affect many different systems in your body and be a cause or consequence of multiple diseases.

Brain and spinal cord: Alzheimer's disease, multiple sclerosis, Parkinson's disease

Thyroid: Thyroiditis

Lungs: Allergies, asthma, COPD, lung cancer

Liver: Chronic hepatitis

Kidneys: Chronic kidney disease, kidney failure, nephritis

Eyes: Macular degeneration, retinal degeneration, uveitis

Heart and blood vessels: Atherosclerosis (hardening of the arteries), heart disease

Pancreas: Type 1 diabetes

Digestive system: Inflammatory bowel disease, including Crohn's disease and ulcerative colitis

Joints: Some forms of arthritis, including rheumatoid arthritis and psoriatic arthritis

Also:

Skin: Acne, eczema, psoriasis, skin cancer

Immune system: Autoimmune disorders such as lupus

without your being aware of it—contributes to some of the nation's leading killers, including cardiovascular disease, cancer, and type 2 diabetes, which are together responsible for about two-thirds of all deaths in the United States.

What makes this type of low-grade inflammation so mysterious and frightening is its silent nature. While a red and swollen cut—or a joint hobbled by an autoimmune disease—is an obvious manifestation, inflammation that lies deep within the body is invisible and insidious. That doesn't mean we are powerless to fight it, however. Both inflammation and the diseases it causes are often preventable with the right combination of lifestyle measures, including a healthful diet, regular exercise, weight control, stress reduction, and smoking cessation.

Of course, it's impossible to draw hard-and-fast rules as to how big a problem this type of inflammation will be for you. How you, your partner, or a child responds to its effects is unique—driven by a combination of genes, lifestyle, and current health. Furthermore, holes still exist in our understanding of inflammation. For many conditions, researchers have not yet fully determined whether inflammation actually causes the disease process, contributes to it (along with other factors), or is an effect of the disease. And

A brief history of inflammation

Inflammation is hardly a new discovery. In the first century, Roman physician Aulus Cornelius Celsus first described the four hallmark signs or "pillars" of inflammation: *rubor* (redness), *tumor* (swelling), *calor* (heat), and *dolor* (pain). This simplistic definition was based on symptoms, rather than an understanding of the deeper physiological processes. Two centuries later, Galen, the physician to Roman emperor Marcus Aurelius, recognized that inflammation was the body's response to injury.

Until the beginning of the 19th century, much of the thinking around inflammation was based on speculation and reasoning, rather than on true science. It wasn't until technological advances enabled scientists to peer through microscopes and witness the actual cellular activities at work during inflammatory reactions that the scientific underpinnings of the process began to emerge. Scientists watched in wonder as white blood cells migrated to the site of the injury or infection, where some started gobbling up germs, while others swept up cellular debris. Biologists postulated that inflammation wasn't a single event, as had been previously assumed, but rather a series of steps that started with an injury to the tissues and ended with their repair.

In 1871, Rudolf Virchow, the German scientist known as the "father of modern pathology," added a fifth sign to Celsus's four: loss of function in the affected area. He described the process of inflammation as a manifestation of disease arising from the release of nutrients from damaged blood vessels, which caused a rush of cells to the site. Virchow was also the first to surmise that, while short-term (acute) inflammation promoted healing, long-term (chronic) inflammation could have damaging implications, including the development of cancer (see "Inflammation and cancer," page 49).

While pathologists studied the ways in which the human body responds to disease and injury, and immunologists investigated how the immune system reacts to foreign invaders, the fledgling pharmaceutical industry of the 19th century began searching for ways to dampen inflammation. Although aspirin had been discovered in the late 1890s and used for joint inflammation, a highlight of drug discovery came in 1962, when Merck researchers identified a rodent model on which they could test potential anti-inflammatory medications. This model dramatically sped up the drug development process and led to the introduction a year later of the nonsteroidal anti-inflammatory drug (NSAID) indomethacin (Indocin), which is still used to treat gout and other inflammatory conditions today. However, the mechanism behind the effects of indomethacin and aspirin remained elusive until the 1970s, when pharmacologist John Vane discovered that these drugs work by blocking the production of pain-promoting hormones called prostaglandins. His finding led to the development of ibuprofen (Advil, Motrin), naproxen (Aleve), and the more than 20 other NSAIDs we now have available to reduce inflammation.

In our time, scientists have also elucidated the role genetics plays in the inflammatory process and the benefits of lifestyle choices like diet and exercise in controlling it. Today, we realize that inflammation encompasses a complex interplay of many different events, by which tissue damage activates signals that launch and perpetuate the immune response to both eliminate the threat and repair damaged tissues. We have tools at our disposal that no other generation has had for understanding and dealing with inflammation.

they don't completely agree whether, or which, anti-inflammatory strategies might effectively prevent it and the diseases to which it's linked. But we do know enough to say what kinds of steps you can take toward an anti-inflammatory lifestyle that will help lessen your chances of developing multiple ailments.

This report will lay out a six-point plan to help you do just that (see the Special Section, "Combating chronic inflammation with lifestyle changes," page 29). It will also explore the role of inflammation in various types of diseases—including autoimmune problems, allergies, heart disease, metabolic problems like diabetes, and even cognitive disorders like Alzheimer's disease. But first, you need to understand the two types of inflammation—acute and chronic.

Acute inflammation

Inflammation comes in two forms—acute (short-term) and chronic (long-term). Acute inflammation is the body's immediate response to an injury or infection. It comes on quickly—usually within minutes—and disappears within days.

Acute inflammation is the reaction that occurs when you stub your toe, cut your finger while chopping vegetables, catch a cold, or fall and break your leg. It is a vital function, triggered when your immune system detects tissue damage or an invading army of germs (see "Act 2: Innate immunity," page 8). Just as it comes on rapidly, it generally dissipates quickly, resolving within a few hours or days.

You can spot acute inflammation near the surface of the body by its telltale five signs: redness, increased heat, swelling, pain, and loss of function. Blood that has been warmed to the body's core temperature rushing up to the normally cool skin surface causes a feeling of warmth and the appearance of redness on the skin. Fluid from the blood vessels that builds up in tissues leads to swelling. Pressure from that fluid buildup and the release of inflammatory chemicals irritates sensitive nerve fibers, causing pain. As a result of this collection of changes, the tissue in the inflamed area may not be able to function as well it should. For example, you may not be able to walk if you have a twisted ankle, or swallow easily if you have a sore throat.

These signs aren't as apparent when the inflammation lies deeper within the body, particularly in areas lacking sensory nerve endings. That's why a cut to the skin, which is filled with nerve endings, is far more painful than lung inflammation (as with a lung infection such as pneumonia), which affects an organ largely lacking in nerve endings.

How acute inflammation develops

When tissue damage occurs, whether from trauma, harmful substances, or a bacterial or viral invasion, your body sends out pro-inflammatory cells to

---

Good germs, bad germs

The immune system has a vested interest in rooting out harmful microbes such as bacteria, viruses, fungi, and parasites, which is why it quickly deploys white blood cells to surround and consume these hostile organisms. There is a good reason for the attack. The diseases they cause can range from something minor like the common cold to a potentially fatal disease such as meningitis.

However, not every germ is bad for you and deserving of destruction. In fact, you have an entire world of microbes living harmoniously with you—on your skin, and inside your digestive system, nose, and other areas of your body. These trillions of beneficial bacteria, known collectively as the microbiome (see "The role of the microbiome in inflammatory diseases," page 24), act a lot like your own cells, breaking down nutrients and synthesizing the vitamins you need to stay healthy, as well as protecting you from more harmful germs.

Some of these microorganisms—like *Bifidobacterium*—actually help to harness damaging inflammation by stimulating the growth of immune cells that control the inflammatory response. The immune system is trained to distinguish these friendly bacteria from harmful ones so that it does not attack the microorganisms that are good for your health.

Researchers have also discovered that a little bit of exposure to both healthful and harmful germs early in life might be a good thing, priming our immune system to respond more effectively to pathogens in the future. In effect, this exposure "teaches" your immune system how to respond to threats, so that it can regulate the inflammatory response and prevent the type of overreaction that can lead to allergies and asthma.

destroy any damaging substances, heal the tissues, and return the affected area to a state of balance. This rapid response results in all of the symptoms you see when you injure yourself.

First, specialized cells in nearby tissue, called mast cells (see "Meet the players: The innate immune system," page 9), send out the emergency call by releasing the chemical histamine. Close to the area of damage, the walls of tiny blood vessels called capillaries contract to minimize blood loss, but soon afterward, they widen (dilate) to bring more blood to the area. This surge of blood makes the injured part of your body swell up and turn red.

Either directly (because of the injury) or indirectly (from the release of chemicals like histamine), the endothelial cells lining the inner surface of the blood vessels first swell up, but then shrink, increasing the space between them. That extra space between cells makes the blood vessels more porous so that fluid, inflammatory proteins, clotting factors, and white blood cells (a large category of specialized cells that scientists call leukocytes) can migrate from the bloodstream into the affected tissue. The collection of cells and fluid that seeps out of the blood vessels is called exudate. At the same time, the blood circulation in the area slows to give immune cells a chance to collect and respond to the threat. The combination of increased fluid entering the tissues and decreased circulation results in swelling.

As fluid builds up inside the tissues, the body's drainage system kicks in. Just as overflowing storm water empties into a sewer drain, excess fluid from the tissues drains away via the body's lymphatic system. Along with this fluid, germs, toxins, and other harmful substances wash away.

Meanwhile, various types of white blood cells are drawn to the site of injury or infection, summoned by chemotaxins (chemicals released by damaged tissues and germs). The first soldiers in this immune army to arrive at the scene are the neutrophils, the most abundant type of white blood cell, which go on the attack. They and certain other white blood cells (together known as phagocytes (see "Meet the players," page 9) engulf, consume, and destroy any harmful organisms. Byproducts of this process, along with continuing distress signals sent out by damaged tissues, magnify the inflammatory response.

> ### Signs of acute inflammation
> - Pain
> - Redness
> - Heat
> - Swelling
> - Immobility or loss of function

As this battle between pathogens and immune cells rages on, it leaves a battlefield strewn with living and dead white blood cells, fluid, germs, and lymphatic fluid, collectively known as pus. The immune system eventually sends out another team of white blood cells, called macrophages, to clean up this refuse of war. But sometimes pus builds up within an empty pocket, forming a swollen area known as an abscess.

How the process subsides

Once the battle is over, the body begins repairing the damage and the subsequent inflammation. Many of the same mechanisms that sprang into action initially now switch gears to cart away dead cells and repair damaged tissue.

A group of fat-based molecules swoops in to prevent further damage and begin the healing process. These specialized pro-resolving mediators, as they are called, help to resolve inflammation and prevent it from getting out of control. These molecules are so efficient that researchers are trying to harness their abilities into treatments for injuries, infections, and chronic inflammatory diseases.

The surviving cells replicate to replace ones that were lost in battle. Cells that are part of less complex structures, such as the surface of the skin, multiply easily. Cells in more complicated organs, such as the liver or glands, do not normally increase in number but may be prompted to do so after damage has occurred. If it is impossible to regrow normal tissue at the site because of the extent of the damage, scar tissue may form.

As the immune system goes back to normal, the redness fades, the swelling goes down, and the pain recedes. The internal and external signs of inflammation dissipate within a few hours or days.

Chronic inflammation

In contrast with acute inflammation, chronic inflammation is not short-lived—and it is rarely helpful. Although it may begin with the same cellular actions as acute inflammation, it morphs into a lingering state that persists for months or years. The body sounds the alarm and emergency help arrives, but the threat never recedes, and the fire continues to burn.

Chronic inflammation is a slower but more insidious process than acute inflammation, and it has been linked to a number of serious diseases, including heart disease, stroke, type 2 diabetes, cancer, Alzheimer's, and arthritis (see Figure 1, page 2).

How acute inflammation turns chronic

In chronic inflammation, what may have started as the solution—for example, as a way to rid the body of a dangerous invader—instead becomes the problem. Chronically inflamed tissues continue to send out alarm signals that trigger the body's immune response, long after the threat has cleared. When white blood cells heed the call and arrive at the scene, they may attack healthy tissues and organs, further amplifying the response and setting up a persistent inflammatory state. As a result, rather than healing the tissues, the body breaks them down further. For example, when pro-inflammatory cells remain in the blood vessels, they promote the buildup of sticky plaque—the same plaque responsible for cardiovascular disease. The body sees this plaque as foreign, and it sends out another army of first responders.

Chronic inflammation can develop in any of several ways. One possibility is that the threat remains because the body can't rid itself of the offending substance, be it an infectious organism, an irritant, or a chemical toxin. The immune system is pretty good at eliminating invaders, but sometimes pathogens resist even our best defenses and hide out in tissues, provoking the inflammatory response again and again. Or, your body can't effectively break down and remove damaging chemicals.

Another possible scenario is that the immune system goes into "threat mode" when no true threat exists. In an autoimmune disorder, the immune system seems to become overly sensitized to the body's own healthy cells and tissue. It reacts against the joints, intestines, or other organs and tissues as if they were dangerous. As the inflammatory response continues, it damages the body instead of healing it.

Unhealthful lifestyle choices, too, can cause ongoing inflammation. Poor habits like smoking, failing to exercise regularly, or eating a diet high in refined carbohydrates can contribute to chronic inflammation over time. This ongoing inflammation is so harmful that the associated diseases—including heart disease, stroke, diabetes, cancer, and chronic obstructive pulmonary disease—are collectively the leading causes of death worldwide. Three out of every five people around the world die from a disease that has been linked to inflammation. It is therefore chronic inflammation that we want to combat with lifestyle interventions, and possibly medications.

Signs and symptoms of chronic inflammation

The symptoms of chronic inflammation may not be as obvious as those of acute inflammation. There may be no sharp twinge of pain as when you cut yourself, no swelling or redness to alert you to a problem. Many of the symptoms are more subtle and are common to other conditions, making it hard to discern what the cause actually is.

Some of the signs and symptoms of chronic inflammation are
- fatigue and lack of energy
- depression, anxiety
- muscle aches and joint pain
- constipation, diarrhea, and other gastrointestinal complaints
- changes in weight or appetite
- headaches
- a "fuzzy" mental state.

Unlike the classic signs of acute inflammation, these symptoms linger over the long term, or they come and go over time. ♥

The biology of the immune response

Before we get into the ways that inflammation can lead to disease, it is helpful to understand a bit about the sophisticated network of cells and molecules that constitute the immune system. This chapter provides some basic explanations that serve as the foundation for the rest of the report. If you are already familiar with this information or you have no interest in the scientific details that underlie the inflammatory mechanisms, feel free to skip this chapter. However, you might find its contents useful, especially for explaining terms that you will encounter in upcoming chapters. (Briefer definitions of these terms appear in the Glossary, page 53.)

The immune response in three acts

Inflammation originates with the immune system—the defensive network that protects you from invading organisms like bacteria, fungi, and viruses, as well as from cancers that arise within our bodies.

The immune response is essentially a sequence of events that occurs after an invader breaches the body's outer defenses or when tissues are damaged in other ways. Each of these events has players with assigned roles. Because timing is key to success, think of the body's immune response as a three-act drama. Act 1 features the arrival of the bad guys (the pathogens) and the body's first attempts to thwart their progress. Act 2 features the players of the innate immune system and their efforts to engulf the invaders and send for reinforcements. Act 3 features the components of the adaptive immune system, which build a defense against repeat attacks. The entire process is enormously complex, but the following summary gives a basic outline.

Act 1: Defending the barricades

The best approach to defeating germs is to bar them from entry in the first place. Your body has a deceptively simple set of initial barriers to keep out unwanted microorganisms—and, in the event they manage to sneak in, strategies to deal with them on the spot.

Skin, the largest organ of the body, is a formidable barrier to infection. Not only does it function as an impressive physical obstacle, but it's also an unfriendly environment for many microbes. The skin's surface is slightly acidic, and some areas are quite dry: neither condition suits many microbes, which prefer moisture and a less acidic environment.

In addition, the skin is already populated by good soldiers: bacteria that call your skin "home," effectively hanging out a "No Trespassing" sign for others. In fact, many parts of your body teem with bacteria. Some are freeloaders, doing nothing but enjoying your hospitality. Others, however, are necessary for the optimal functioning of the body. Without the helpful bacteria on the skin, for example, infectious microbes would have easier access.

Impressive though it is, the skin can't provide perfect protection. It has openings through which food, water, air, and other substances enter or leave the body. The eyes, mouth, ears, airways, digestive tract, and urogenital tract are examples of the body's gateways. Although vital, they provide a way for pathogens to slip in.

Not surprisingly, the body is on the lookout for pathogens, and it mounts regular surveillance to eliminate them before they have time to establish themselves. For example, the conjunctiva (the mucous membrane that covers the outside of the eyes) is periodically moistened and swept, like the windshield of a car. The high acid level inside the stomach kills many dangerous bacteria, as do the beneficial bacteria in the digestive tract, which keep disease-causing bacteria under control most of the time. Mucosa (the soft tissues that line various tracts) also have antimicrobial properties. But sometimes these responses aren't enough. Then it's time to bring in the Act 2 players.

Act 2: Innate immunity

Innate immunity is the next line of defense after the barriers of the skin and mucosa are breached. The role of the innate immune system is to attack invading pathogens, triggering an immediate inflammatory response and firing up the third line of defense, the adaptive immune system. Innate immunity got its name because everyone is born with it—it is innate.

Innate immunity is nonspecialized, meaning that it is not specifically targeted at a particular virus or bacterium. This is how it can mount such a quick response. Compare that to adaptive immunity, which needs time to develop in the early years of life. Innate immunity is the body's first *active* response to specific pathogens.

The innate immune system has a multipronged response (see Figure 2, below left).

Engulfing the invader. The innate immune system is best known for a category of white blood cells called phagocytes, which reside very close to the layer of epithelial cells that line much of the body's surface. Phagocytic cells, such as neutrophils, macrophages, and dendritic cells, destroy pathogens by engulfing them and chemically chewing them up (see "Meet the players: The innate immune system," page 9).

Sending alerts for the adaptive immune system. After a phagocyte engulfs an invading microbe, it displays pieces of protein from the microbe (antigens) on its surface. This alerts the adaptive immune system to the invader and activates other immune cells called T cells, so they can recognize an infected cell in the body and prepare for battle (see "Act 3: Adaptive immunity," page 9).

Yet that is not enough to trigger the full adaptive immune response. There also needs to be a danger signal or flag displayed on the surface of the phagocyte to fully rouse the adaptive immune system into action. This process begins with proteins in the phagocytes called pattern recognition receptors (PRRs). PRRs enable the phagocyte to quickly distinguish unique molecular patterns—appropriately named "alarmins"—in bacteria and other pathogens as well as in damaged body tissues. Alarmins come in two forms:

- Pathogen-associated molecular patterns (PAMPs) are unique molecules found in germs like bacteria and viruses, but not in humans.
- Damage-associated molecular patterns (DAMPs) are molecules released by human cells when tissue has been injured or transformed (such as by a tumor, trauma, or lack of oxygen).

Both PAMPs and DAMPs bind to receptors on immune cells, similar to the way that a key fits into a lock. Binding activates a cascade of signals that mobilize an army of immune cells to both attack the

Figure 2: Innate immune system

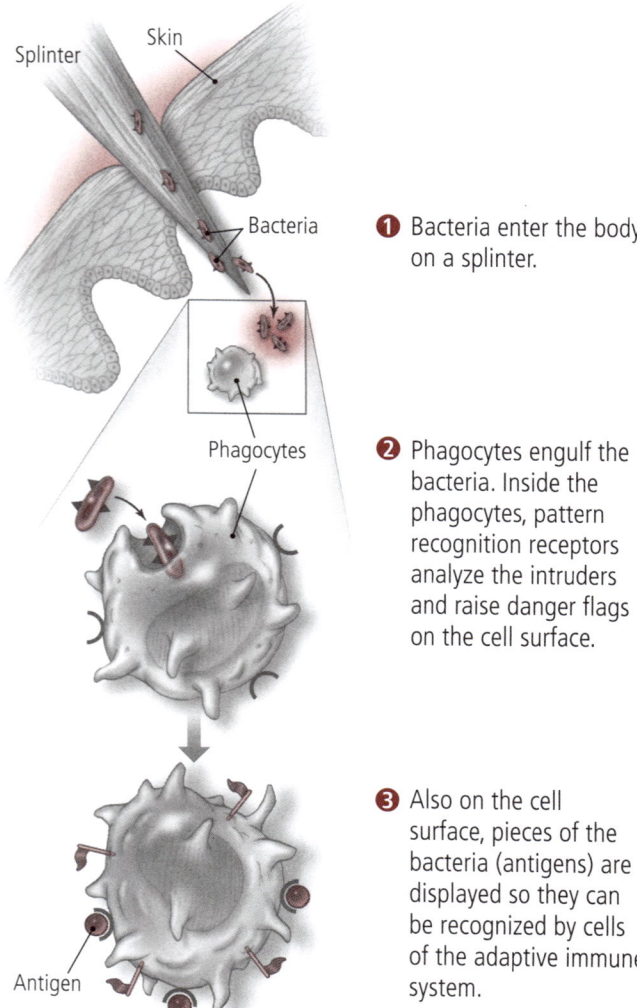

1. Bacteria enter the body on a splinter.

2. Phagocytes engulf the bacteria. Inside the phagocytes, pattern recognition receptors analyze the intruders and raise danger flags on the cell surface.

3. Also on the cell surface, pieces of the bacteria (antigens) are displayed so they can be recognized by cells of the adaptive immune system.

The innate immune cells known as phagocytes attack germs by chewing them up and displaying pieces of them on their surfaces along with a danger flag as a signal for help.

invader and set off more alarm signals. Immune cells then either directly engulf and destroy the invaders, as described above, or generate other substances to destroy them.

Unleashing interferons. Yet another strategy of the innate immune system involves the presence of virus-detecting proteins inside cells. The detection of a virus causes the cell to release antiviral proteins known as interferons, which attach themselves to neighboring uninfected cells, thus making them resistant to the virus. The name provides the clue to function: interferons interfere with the viral advance.

Marking for destruction. Blood also participates in innate immunity. Proteins known as complement proteins circulate in the blood, coating invading bugs and punching holes in them to destroy them. Small fragments of complement proteins also adhere to the pathogen surface, flagging them for destruction by phagocytes.

In sum, the innate immune system is a necessary rapid-response system, but it has a few limitations. Although PRRs can recognize many kinds of pathogens, they are less effective against certain others. Second, the innate immune system retains no memory of the foe it vanquished. That's why the adaptive immune response is so important.

Act 3: Adaptive immunity

Adaptive immunity is a more gradual process by which white blood cells called lymphocytes are primed to distinguish foes from the body's own cells. (Autoimmune diseases result when this process goes awry.)

Meet the players: The innate immune system

All of these immune cells play a part in the innate immune system response. A number of them—such as basophils, cytokines, dendritic cells, and mast cells—are directly linked to inflammation.

Basophils are a type of white blood cell and part of a group known as granulocytes. Inside these cells are small particles (granules) containing enzymes that break down the proteins inside bacteria and fungi. Basophils release the chemical histamine, which makes small blood vessels dilate and become a bit porous, allowing white blood cells and proteins to leave the circulation to attack invaders.

Chemokines are a family of cytokines (see below) that attract white blood cells to the site of an infection or damage.

Cytokines are signaling proteins that immune cells release to orchestrate the inflammatory response. They include interferons, interleukins, and tumor necrosis factor, among others.

Dendritic cells are the immune system's sentinels. During an active attack, they recognize and ingest foreign antigens, and they produce pro-inflammatory cytokines that enhance the innate immune response. They also serve as a bridge to the adaptive immune system, by traveling through the bloodstream to the lymph nodes and spleen, where they expose cells of the adaptive immune system to the antigens they've ingested, essentially "teaching" these immune cells to respond to future threats.

Eosinophils are a type of white blood cell, also in the group known as granulocytes (see "Basophils," above). They secrete toxic substances that kill bacteria, viruses, and parasites. The immune system carefully controls eosinophil release, because these cells can be highly damaging to healthy tissues, such as the heart, nerves, or skin.

Macrophages are the gluttonous eaters that leave the bloodstream and arrive at the site of an infection or injury to disinfect and clean up. They eat up bacteria and other pathogens, along with dead cells and other debris damaged tissue leaves behind. Macrophages also release cytokines to recruit other white blood cells.

Mast cells are immune cells present in connective tissue. They initiate the inflammatory response by releasing cytokines and pro-inflammatory chemicals like histamine, which is a key feature of allergic reactions. Histamine increases blood flow to the area by causing the blood vessels to dilate (widen).

Neutrophils are white blood cells that are part of the body's frontline defense. In part, this is because you have so many of them circulating in your bloodstream. A healthy adult makes about 100 billion neutrophils each day. They are also a type of granulocyte (see "Basophils," above left). Neutrophils are also classified as phagocytes; they arrive within minutes of the pathogen attack or injury and begin to engulf and destroy the germs.

Phagocytes are a category of immune cells that serve as the scavengers of the immune system. The types of white blood cells that are classified as phagocytes include neutrophils, monocytes, macrophages, and dendritic cells. They patrol the bloodstream looking for viruses and other pathogens, and are summoned to the scene of injury or infection by chemicals called cytokines.

If the first line of active defense—the innate immune response—is unsuccessful at vanquishing the foe within about four to seven days, the second line of active defense, adaptive immunity, swings into action.

Adaptive immunity is a slower process than innate immunity, but it is far more precise (see Table 1, at right). It recognizes pathogens and targets them specifically. The adaptive immune system produces "memory" cells that enable it to remember antigens and respond again to them in the future. That's why, once you get a disease like chickenpox, you are said to be "immune" to it. If you are exposed again to the varicella zoster virus, which causes chickenpox, your immune system will automatically know to fight it off.

How the adaptive immune system responds to a threat depends on where that threat is—already in your cells (cell-mediated responses), or in your blood and body fluids (antibody responses).

T cells carry out cell-mediated responses. T cells are lymphocytes, a type of white blood cell produced in bone marrow. While still immature, they travel to a small organ behind your breastbone known as the thymus (hence, the "T" in "T cell"). There, they are "trained" to distinguish foreign antigens from the body's own antigens (self-antigens). Once mature, T cells leave the thymus; many are stored in the lymph nodes, spleen, tonsils, appendix, and small intestine, while others circulate through the bloodstream and lymphatic system, on the prowl for invaders.

T cells can recognize infected cells in one of two ways—either by seeing antigens (proteins) from germs

Table 1: Differences between innate and adaptive immunity

INNATE IMMUNITY	ADAPTIVE IMMUNITY
Responds fast (within hours)	Responds slower (in days)
Involves phagocytes (macrophages, dendritic cells, and neutrophils)	Involves lymphocytes (T cells and B cells)
Recognizes general patterns of pathogens	Recognizes specific pathogens

Figure 3: Adaptive immune response: T cells

T cells attack and destroy invaders, then multiply to prepare for a future invasion of the same germ.

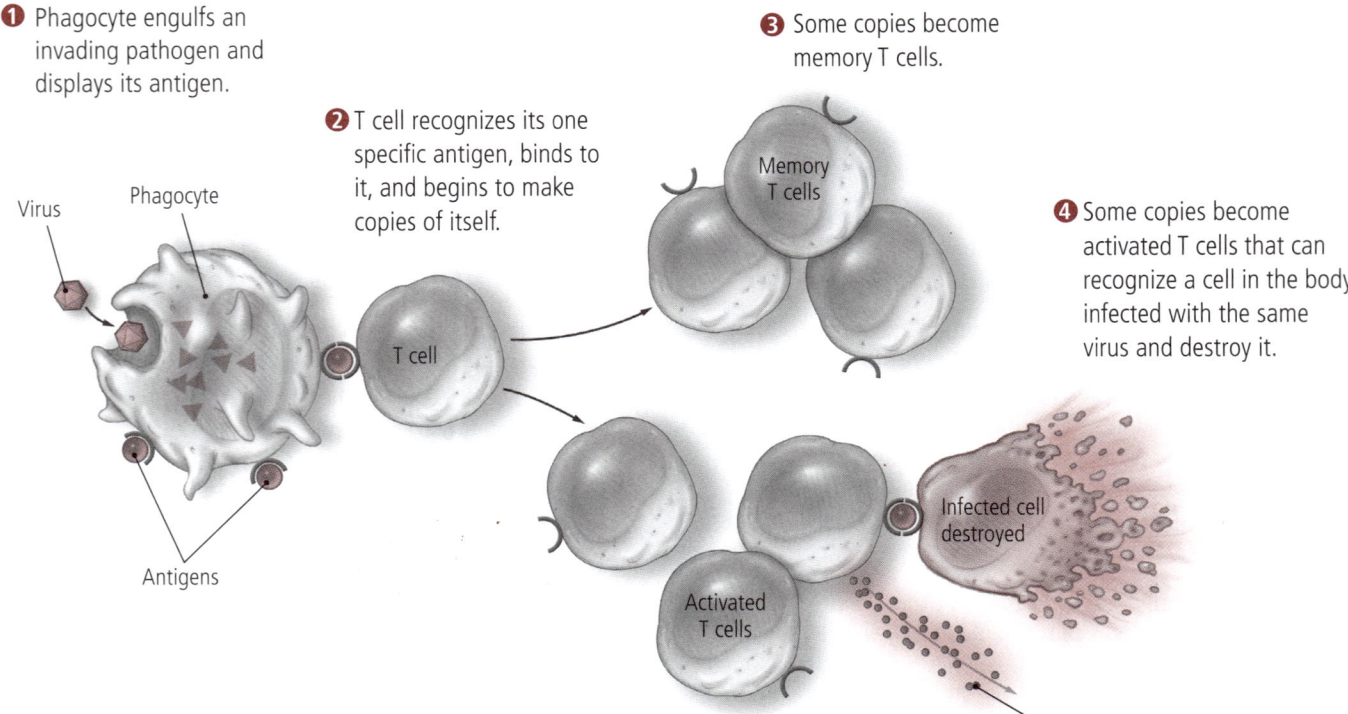

❶ Phagocyte engulfs an invading pathogen and displays its antigen.

❷ T cell recognizes its one specific antigen, binds to it, and begins to make copies of itself.

❸ Some copies become memory T cells.

❹ Some copies become activated T cells that can recognize a cell in the body infected with the same virus and destroy it.

Figure 4: Adaptive immune response: B cells

B cells produce antibodies to block invaders and multiply to prepare for future invasions of the same pathogen.

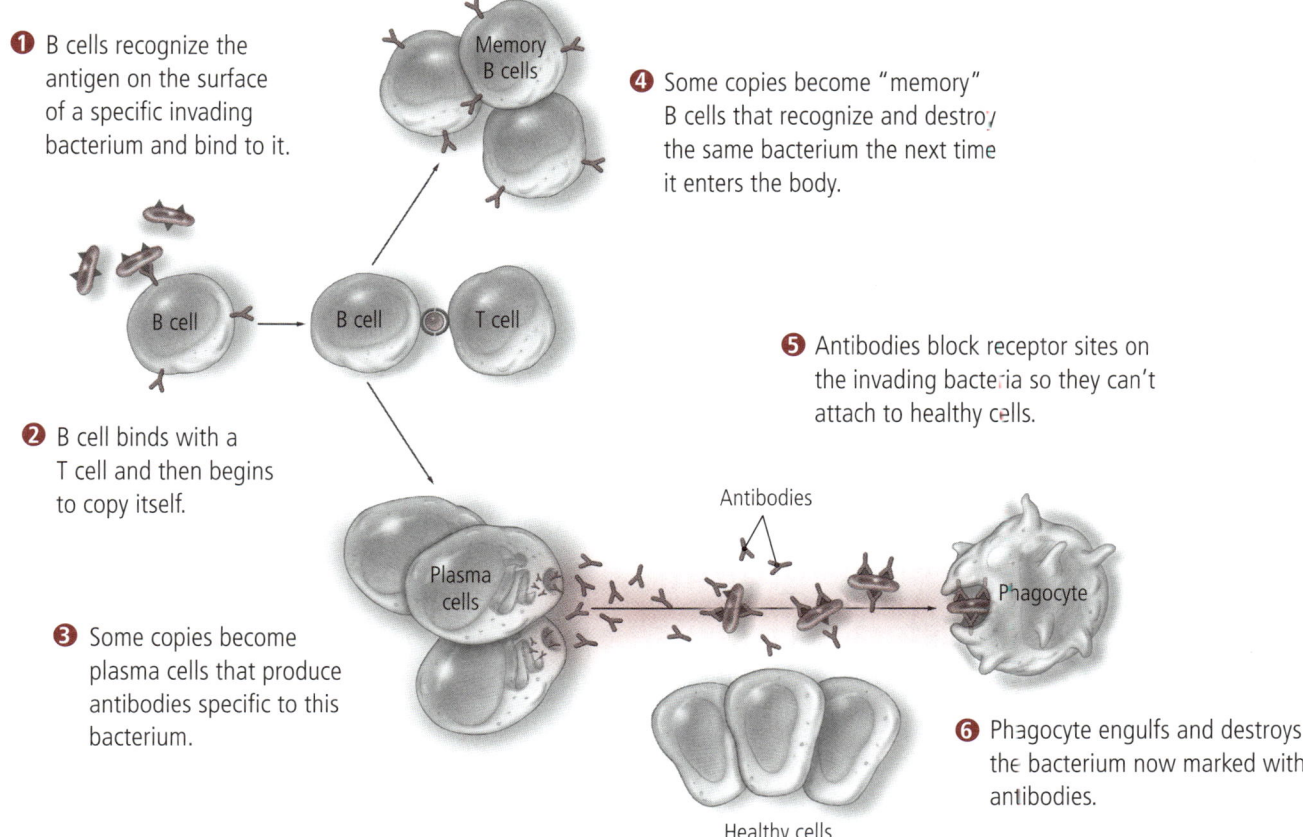

❶ B cells recognize the antigen on the surface of a specific invading bacterium and bind to it.

❷ B cell binds with a T cell and then begins to copy itself.

❸ Some copies become plasma cells that produce antibodies specific to this bacterium.

❹ Some copies become "memory" B cells that recognize and destroy the same bacterium the next time it enters the body.

❺ Antibodies block receptor sites on the invading bacteria so they can't attach to healthy cells.

❻ Phagocyte engulfs and destroys the bacterium now marked with antibodies.

they have encountered before or by identifying antigens that the innate immune system has tagged for them (see Figure 3, page 10). When T cells recognize a foreign entity, they develop further into any of four specialized variations:

- Helper T cells help other immune cells work more effectively. There are several subtypes of helper T cells. Th1 cells are vital to controlling certain kinds of viral and bacterial infections. Th2 cells promote the production of antibodies by B cells. In an allergic reaction, however, Th2 cells may respond to substances that are not actually harmful.
- Killer T cells attach to antigens on infected or cancerous cells, make holes in the cell membrane, and then inject enzymes that destroy the cell.
- Regulatory T cells produce substances that regulate the immune response, preventing it from continuing unchecked or damaging the body's tissues. These cells also help distinguish between the body's own cells and invaders.
- Memory T cells remember antigens of particular germs, so they can identify them in the future.

B cells carry out antibody responses. B cells produce antibodies—proteins that target specific antigens. They can remember an almost infinite number of different antigens. When an antibody from a B cell recognizes and binds to an antigen on an invading virus particle, bacterium, or other pathogen, it inactivates the invader by preventing it from binding to receptors on body cells. The binding process also marks these invaders for destruction by other immune cells (see Figure 4, above).

When good inflammation turns bad

As the previous chapters have explained, inflammation is a key part of the immune response. But this process, which is supposed to save your life, can end up harming you under various circumstances—if the immune response (with its accompanying inflammation) comes on too strong; if it fails to turn off after an infection goes away; if it misfires, causing either allergies or autoimmune disorders; or if it is continually triggered by lifestyle factors. This chapter provides an overview of what goes wrong in each of these cases and the problems that can result. Later chapters will take a closer look at some of those problems.

When the immune system overreacts

The response against harmful germs, or pathogens, is tightly regulated. A set of "brakes" is in place to prevent the immune system from overreacting and producing uncontrolled inflammation, but it is not perfect. If a bacterium, virus, or other pathogen is particularly virulent, or if the immune reaction is especially robust, the inflammatory response may inflict more cell injury than the offending organism itself. For example, a faulty immune system response to a viral infection can cause the immune system to mistakenly attack healthy cells in the brain, leading to life-threatening inflammation called encephalitis.

Another example is acute respiratory distress syndrome (ARDS). People develop ARDS after a severe trauma that either directly or indirectly affects their lungs—for example, when they nearly drown, when they breathe in smoke from a fire, or when they develop a severe case of pneumonia. In ARDS, the body's inflammatory response sends immune cells rushing to the lungs. These immune cells cause tiny blood vessels in the area to leak fluid, as is normal during this reaction. But when fluid leaks into the lungs, it builds up in the alveoli, the air sacs through which oxygen normally passes into the bloodstream. The fluid buildup prevents oxygen from getting into the blood, making it hard to breathe. Without good supportive care, ARDS can be fatal.

The lethal nature of the 1918 flu (which killed an estimated 50 million people worldwide) reflected not only to its ability to replicate quickly and spread easily from person to person, but also to its capacity to provoke ARDS. A flood of immune cells and inflammatory substances quickly overloaded people's bodies and caused fluid to build up in their lungs. In essence, the victims drowned inside their own bodies. This catastrophic inflammatory response was why even young, healthy adults succumbed to the virus. More recently, a version of ARDS appears to have killed many of those who have died from COVID-19.

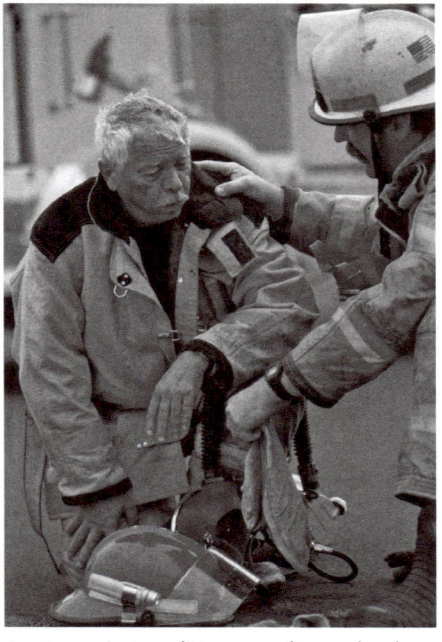

Acute respiratory distress syndrome develops after a trauma—such as a near drowning, smoke from a fire, or a severe lung infection. It involves massive inflammation in the lungs.

Some people are at greater risk than others for a dangerous inflammatory reaction. For example, those with the rare condition hemophagocytic lymphohistiocytosis produce too many activated immune cells. While the cause of this condition is often uncertain, it can be due to an inherited gene mutation, a faulty response to an infection, or a complication of an autoimmune disease such as juvenile rheumatoid arthritis.

When the immune system fails to revert to normal

An essential aspect of an adaptive immune response is the return to a normal or baseline state. Logically, an immune response should wane over time because the only purpose of the activity is to eliminate an antigen or help repair tissue damage. Once the problem that triggered the immune response is gone, the drama is over. Most players leave the stage.

But this does not always happen. Instead, inflammation can simmer on at a low-grade level and become chronic. There are a number of scenarios in which this can happen.

Sometimes the immune system eliminates a threat, but white blood cells continue to attack anyway. With no real enemy left to vanquish, these cells instead destroy healthy tissue in places like the joints, arteries, intestines, or brain. A good example of this is a condition called reactive arthritis, in which an infection (such as one in the intestinal tract) triggers inflammation in the eyes, joints, and urinary tract, even though the infection is gone. Doctors do not know why the immune system behaves this way, although a common theory is "molecular mimicry" (see "Autoimmunity," at right).

In other cases, an infection may be difficult for the immune system to eradicate, so the fight continues. This is what happens in conditions like hepatitis C or HIV. In both cases, the ongoing inflammatory response may cause more damage to the body than the organism itself.

In a third set of cases, the inflammation is prompted not by a germ, but by repeated toxin exposure or a tumor.

When the immune system misfires

The immune system is generally able to perform the tricky task of distinguishing threats from non-threats. For example, most of the time, it knows not to attack food or food components, even though these are "foreign" substances that come from outside the body. But sometimes the system misfires. Allergic reactions develop against things like pollen that pose no danger of infecting cells. Worse, the immune system can go awry and target the body's own tissues, causing a variety of autoimmune conditions.

Hypersensitivity/allergic reactions. Sometimes the immune system develops a sensitivity to otherwise harmless environmental substances such as dust, pollen, shellfish, or pet dander, causing it to misdirect its fire and leading to inflammation (see "Inflammation and allergic responses: When your body rebels against its environment," page 17). During an allergic reaction, the offending substance triggers the immune system to produce a protein called immunoglobulin E (IgE), which travels to mast cells and causes them to release chemicals that set off symptoms like sneezing, itching, swelling, and mucus release. In addition to allergies, hypersensitivity reactions include atopic dermatitis (eczema) and asthma. In some cases, a rapid and very severe reaction called anaphylaxis occurs, which can be deadly if not treated quickly.

Autoimmunity. During hypersensitivity or allergic reactions, the body is responding to external threats. In autoimmune conditions, the perceived enemy comes from within, as the body's defense system mistakenly wages war on your own tissues (see "Inflammation and autoimmune disease: When your body fights itself," page 23).

The reasons autoimmunity develops are complex and not fully understood. Genes clearly play a role; autoimmune diseases such as multiple sclerosis, lupus, and rheumatoid arthritis run in families, and people who have one autoimmune disease are more susceptible to others. Two genes in particular have been identified as increasing the risk for celiac disease, in which the immune system takes aim at the protein gluten in wheat, rye, and barley, but ends up damaging the lining of the small intestine in the process. As a result, the body loses its ability to absorb certain nutrients, leading to osteoporosis, infertility, and a host of other problems.

One theory is that autoimmunity may be the collateral damage of a normal immune response against infection. The idea is that healthy cells like those in the joints or skin can get caught up in the body's response, leading to conditions like rheumatoid arthritis or psoriasis. In some cases, a feat of cellular trickery, known as molecular mimicry, may be involved. Certain bacteria and viruses produce antigens that mimic the body's own proteins. These pathogens still trigger the inflammatory signals that call in the immune response. But because they look like the body's own cells, the immune system begins to see its own cells as foreign. The process leads to the production of autoantibodies—that is, antibodies against self. In a certain subgroup of people, this process can lead to autoimmune diseases—although not everyone with autoantibodies develops an autoimmune disease. It has long been hypothesized that conditions such as rheumatoid arthritis and lupus might be caused by an abnormal immune response to an infectious agent—however, this remains speculation as no infectious cause has ever been found. In fact, the causes of most autoimmune conditions are unknown.

When inflammation is the result of lifestyle or aging

Increasingly, scientists are finding that a number of major diseases involve low-grade chronic inflammation (see "Inflammation and your heart," page 38, "Inflammation and your brain," page 41, "Inflammation and metabolic disease," page 46, and "Inflammation and cancer," page 49). The causes of this inflammation seem related not to infections or autoimmunity, but to factors like a poor diet, advancing age, obesity, a sedentary lifestyle, and stress. Unfortunately, the triggers don't simply go away over time—by definition, lifestyle is the way you live, day in and day out—and that means the inflammation doesn't go away either. Researchers still have much to learn about the causes of low-grade chronic inflammation, but certain problems are coming into clearer focus.

Aging. Chronic inflammation is a risk factor for a number of diseases that become more common with age—including high blood pressure, diabetes, atherosclerosis (hardening of the arteries), and cancer. Yet age itself is associated with higher levels of inflammatory molecules, which leads to a persistent state of low-grade inflammation. Seniors tend to have higher levels of inflammatory cytokines (see "The biology of the immune response," page 7) in their blood than do younger adults. Scientists have dubbed this age-related chronic, low-grade inflammation "inflammaging."

The process by which aging leads to inflammation is highly complex, involving a number of different cellular processes. Among the most important players are molecules called reactive oxygen species (ROS), which include free radicals. ROS molecules contain an oxygen atom with an unpaired electron on their shell. They form during the process of cellular reactions that use oxygen, as well as from environmental exposures such as smoking, drugs, sunlight, or pollution. In order to be stable, an atom must contain a balanced number of negatively charged particles, or electrons, on its outer shell. When the number is unbalanced, the atom will either steal an electron from a nearby molecule, or lose an electron in an attempt to stabilize itself. When one ROS molecule steals an electron, the molecule it stole the electron from then steals an electron, and so on, in a domino-like chain reaction that over time leaves cells damaged. The processes needed to rid the body of these damaged cells create a constant state of inflammation, and as you age, damage accumulates from ROS and its accompanying inflammation.

Also to blame for inflammation in the elderly is the gradual decline of the immune system with age, a process that researchers call immunosenescence. Although the body tries to counteract the damage inflicted by free radicals, eventually it is unable to keep up. Years of accumulated damage take their toll on immune cells. At the same time, the thymus—the tiny organ in the chest where T cells are "trained"—shrinks with age. The result is an overall decline or impairment of immune regulation. The body continues to be exposed to threats (antigens), but it can no longer respond to them as effectively as it once did. Because other parts of the immune system may not be functioning optimally with age, inflammatory molecules may be in a state of constant activation, which leads to low-grade inflammation.

Finally, time takes its toll in the form of extended exposures to harmful substances. The longer you're around, the more you're exposed to damaging pollution, UV radiation from the sun, and the chemicals in cigarettes (if you smoke or spend time near smokers).

Obesity. As the years accumulate, weight tends to accumulate as well —an average of a pound or two a year from early adulthood through middle age. Nearly 40% of Americans are obese (meaning their body mass index is 30 or higher), and inflammation is one of the consequences. The buildup of fat ramps up the immune response, leading to a cycle of constant low-level inflammation.

People who are obese have an excess of adipose tissue, the type of tissue used to store fat. Their fat cells, called adipocytes, are also larger than normal. Fat cells were once thought to be inert storage depots for fatty acids from the diet, but scientists now know this is not the case. Research has revealed that adipocytes produce pro-inflammatory signaling proteins called adipocytokines, which send the immune system into a constant state of alert. As these fat cells grow in size and number, they produce even more adipocytokines. Therefore, the more a person weighs, the more inflammatory substances they produce.

Diet. Food does more than simply nourish your body. How you fill your plate can either promote or help control inflammation. Diets high in saturated fats and refined sugars are associated with the increased production of pro-inflammatory molecules.

Certain foods in particular are known to promote inflammation, including white flour–based carbohydrates (white bread, cookies, cakes, pastries), fried foods, soda and other sugar-sweetened drinks, red and processed meats, margarine, and shortening. Not only do these types of foods directly stimulate the release of inflammatory cytokines, but they also promote weight gain, meaning that there is more fat tissue releasing adipocytokines.

Foods like green leafy vegetables, fatty fish, and olive oil have the opposite effect, suppressing the production of pro-inflammatory molecules and enhancing the production of anti-inflammatory ones (see "Eat to beat inflammation," page 29).

Sedentary lifestyle. The couch potato lifestyle has been linked to a number of health risks, among

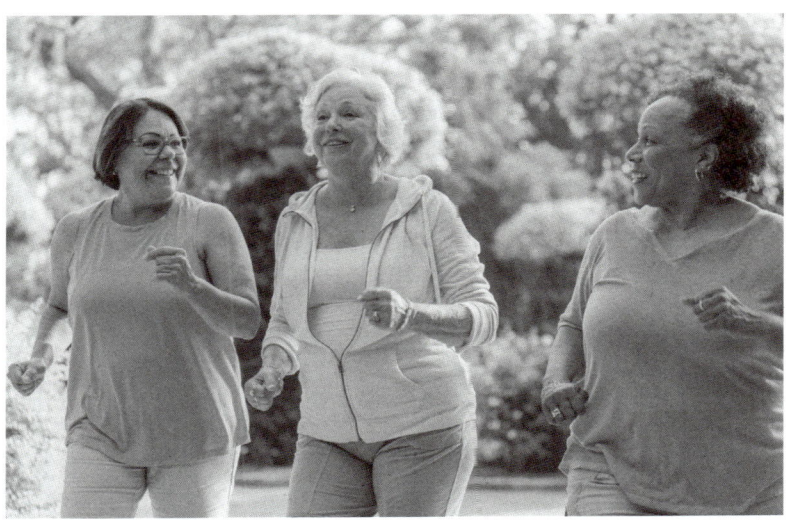

Chronic inflammation is linked to many lifestyle factors, which by definition do not go away, because they're part of our lifestyles. But most are in our power to change, including excess weight, a poor diet, sedentary behavior, and smoking.

them obesity, high blood pressure, heart disease, type 2 diabetes, osteoporosis, and depression. Several studies have also associated a sedentary way of life with increased inflammation. In much of the research, it's been hard to tease out whether inflammation is the direct result of sitting too much, or whether it comes from problems that are often part and parcel of a sedentary lifestyle, such as obesity, high blood sugar, or a poor diet. But a study in the journal *PLOS One* found elevated levels of the pro-inflammatory cytokine interleukin-6 (IL-6) in people who spent a lot of time sitting, even after the researchers adjusted for these related factors. This finding suggests that a sedentary lifestyle may have a direct effect on inflammation, underscoring the need to get up and move around throughout the day.

Smoking. Beyond its contributions to cancer, lung disease, and a host of other health problems, smoking is a known accelerator of inflammation. The action of lighting the end of a cigarette generates a witches' brew made up of thousands of chemicals, many of which are toxic to human cells and tissues. Burning tobacco generates ROS, which damage the cells of the airways. ROS and other components of tobacco smoke, as well as damaged airway cells, send out signals that activate the inflammatory response. In the airways of regular smokers, this produces a state of constant injury and inflammation. The good news is that quitting smok-

Hormones and inflammation

The immune system works closely with the endocrine system—the collection of glands that release hormones that control metabolism, growth, and other functions throughout the body. Steroid hormones, which include sex hormones (like estrogen, progesterone, and testosterone) and the glucocorticoids, help modulate the immune system response.

Glucocorticoids, a group of hormones that includes cortisol, are part of the immune system's feedback mechanism. These hormones help regulate inflammation during the elimination of pathogens and the repair of tissues following an illness or injury. Glucocorticoids have such powerful anti-inflammatory properties that synthetic versions of them (cortisone, hydrocortisone, prednisone) are mainstays in the treatment of inflammatory diseases like rheumatoid arthritis.

Sex hormones affect inflammation too, but in different ways. Male hormones (androgens) like testosterone are primarily anti-inflammatory, whereas female hormones (such as estrogen and progesterone) can either suppress or promote inflammation. These differences may underlie the stronger immune responses women mount, against both foreign agents and their own bodies. This could help explain, at least in part, why women are at much higher risk than men for most autoimmune diseases.

---

ing can help reverse this process. Within a few years after a person stops smoking, blood levels of C-reactive protein (CRP) and other markers of inflammation drop.

Even though cigarette smoke promotes inflammation in general, it actually dampens the innate immune response needed to protect you against infections and cancer. For example, when airway cells that have been exposed to tobacco smoke are infected with the influenza virus, they produce lower levels of pro-inflammatory cytokines like IL-6 and interleukin-8 than do cells that have not been exposed to smoke, which allows the virus to replicate unchecked. The effects of smoking on immune function may be why smokers are more likely to develop tuberculosis and why the flu and pneumonia tend to be more severe among smokers.

Stress. Stress is similar to inflammation in that it can be helpful in small amounts, but detrimental when allowed to continue long-term. A certain amount of stress helps you succeed, pushing you to study hard for a test or meet a deadline at work. But too much of it can damage your health.

The body has evolved an emergency stress response system, called the fight-or-flight response, to help you survive threats like a bear about to pounce or a motorcycle speeding toward you. The release of stress hormones like cortisol (see "Hormones and inflammation," at left) and adrenaline makes your heart beat faster, your breath quicken, and your muscles prepare for action. That is all well and good when you are under threat, but if this response fires again and again because of a stressful job or an unhappy marriage, these powerful reactions continue to occur when no real threat is present.

The continuous rush of cortisol eventually makes your tissues and immune cells less sensitive to its effects. As a result, cortisol becomes less effective at regulating the inflammatory response, and inflammation can spiral out of control.

Inflammation and allergic responses: When your body rebels against its environment

More than 50 million Americans are allergic to something normally innocuous, such as dust, pollen, pets' dander, eggs, shellfish, or mold. Exposure to such a trigger brings a wave of misery, with symptoms like sneezing, runny eyes, or (in more severe cases) hives, swollen lips, and wheezing. The most extreme of these reactions, known as anaphylaxis, is a bodywide response that can be deadly.

The term "allergy," which comes from the Greek word for "other," was first coined in 1906 by Austrian pediatrician Clemens von Pirquet. He used the word to describe the abnormal immune system reaction, or hypersensitivity response, triggered by a foreign substance that he termed an "allergen."

The hypersensitivity disorders produced by this overreaction include allergic rhinitis (colloquially termed "hay fever"), allergic asthma, anaphylaxis, atopic dermatitis (eczema), and food allergies. Allergies, asthma, and eczema often occur together, launched by the same substances that set off allergy symptoms.

Allergies

In certain people, the immune system responds to harmless substances like pollen or animal dander as if they were dangerous infectious agents. Genes are partly responsible. But as the incidence of allergies has risen in the developed world—in tandem with a reduction in infectious diseases—the so-called hygiene hypothesis has also gained traction. Proposed by immunologist David Strachan in the 1980s, it holds that exposure to germs early in life "trains" a child's fledgling immune system to identify disease-causing pathogens by stimulating T cells (see "T cells carry out cell-mediated responses," page 10)—and that without exposure to the true "bad guys" in early childhood, certain components of the immune system don't develop properly. The result is an allergy, as cells of the immune system that normally help fend off invading viruses and bacteria become overactive and target these noninfectious substances.

Eating, inhaling, or touching any of these substances can trigger an allergic reaction in people who are sensitive to them. The most common allergens include

- grass and tree pollen
- animal dander (shed pieces of skin and fur)
- dust mites
- latex
- foods such as peanuts, tree nuts, fish, shellfish, eggs, and milk
- insect venom.

To become allergic to one of these substances, the body needs to undergo a process called sensitization

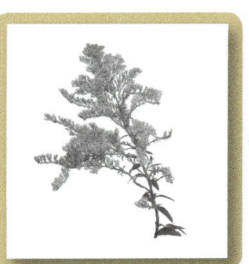 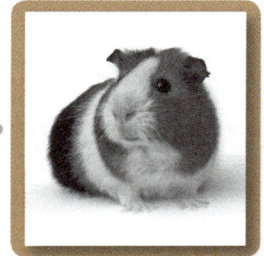 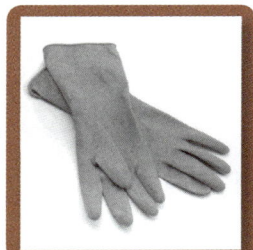 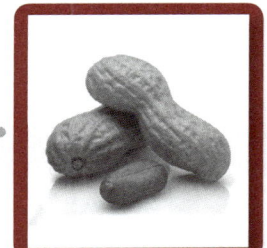 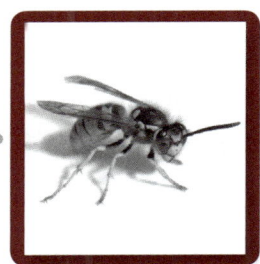

Normally, the immune system can distinguish between harmful substances like germs and harmless ones such as pollen or animal dander. But in people with allergies, the immune system targets innocuous substances.

(see Figure 5, page 19). When allergens enter the body, immune cells called antigen-presenting cells (such as dendritic cells) capture them, and, as the name implies, present them to other immune cells, particularly T cells.

There are two types of T cells: Th1 and Th2. During a normal reaction, Th1 cells release cytokines that cause B cells to start manufacturing a type of protective antibody called immunoglobulin G (IgG). Antibodies are proteins the immune system produces when it perceives a potential threat. The body makes five immunoglobulins: IgA, IgD, IgE, IgG, and IgM. IgG antibodies circulate throughout the bloodstream and go after bacteria, viruses, and other harmful organisms.

Th2 cells also direct B cells to produce antibodies, but the IgE kind. IgE primes the immune system to recognize the allergen the next time it enters the body. This process is known as sensitization. IgE binds to receptors on the surface of mast cells in the tissues and basophils in the bloodstream. A single exposure to the offending substance provokes an acute (early-phase) reaction, which doesn't produce symptoms, but it readies the immune system to be on the lookout for that allergen in the future.

The next time that person is exposed to the same allergen, IgE is able to bind to it. Within minutes of the allergen exposure, another early-phase reaction is set into motion. Binding causes the mast cell or basophil to release chemicals like histamine, prostaglandins, and leukotrienes that produce inflammation. The release of these chemicals leads to some or all of the hallmark symptoms of an allergic reaction:

- widening of the blood vessels, which produces reddened skin or eyes, or both
- leaking of the blood vessels, causing swelling of the tissues and tearing of the eyes
- contraction of muscles in the lungs, causing wheezing and difficulty breathing
- increased mucus secretion, producing a runny nose
- stimulation of sensory nerves, causing sneezing, coughing, and itching.

The chemicals that mast cells release attract other white blood cells—eosinophils, neutrophils, and basophils—to the area. This part of the allergic response is known as the late-phase reaction, and it occurs hours after exposure to the allergen. These white blood cells essentially move into the tissues and remain there.

Both the mast cells and the recruited white blood cells release chemicals called cytokines that damage tissues. When exposure to the allergen is continuous or repeated, it causes persistent inflammation, along with changes to cells in the area that can permanently reshape the structure and function of the affected organ. For example, people with chronic asthma can develop additional mucus-producing cells in their airways, and more of the smooth muscle cells that cause the muscles of the airway to thicken.

Eczema

Eczema, also known as atopic dermatitis, is an inflammatory skin disease that produces patches of red, intensely itchy skin. It often begins in infancy, but it can last into adolescence and adulthood. Although the condition is generally considered more annoying than dangerous, it may increase the risk of heart disease and stroke, possibly because of increased inflammation in the body. Eczema can also lead to skin infections, since the skin's barrier function is impaired.

Both genetics and the environment play roles in the development of eczema. People with eczema have high blood levels of IgE antibodies, which are associated

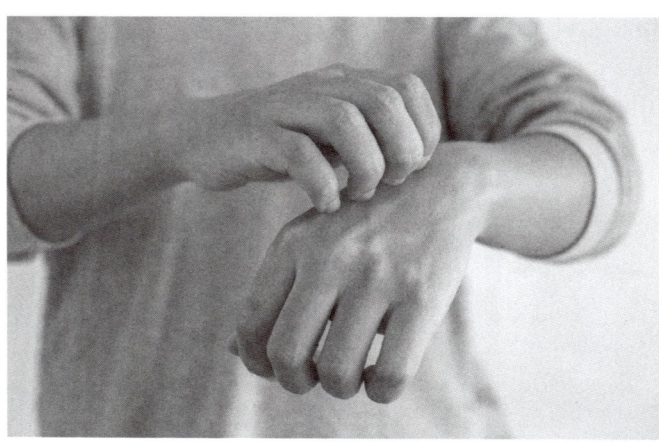

Eczema produces patches of red, intensely itchy skin. The skin reaction is the result of an abnormal immune response that produces inflammation inside the body.

Continued on page 20

Figure 5: Developing an allergy: A two-step process

1. First exposure (sensitization): You produce antibodies that will recognize the allergen in the future.

Dendritic cells, a type of immune cell that monitors the body tissues for allergens and other foreign materials, begin the innate immune response. These cells recognize an allergen as an invader, gobbling it up from wherever it landed (the lining of your nose, for example). They process the invader and display a recognizable portion as an antigen, which activates a special type of T cell called Tfh (follicular helper T). This sets off a complex chain reaction involving the release of cytokines, chemicals that signal B cells to produce IgE antibodies; these antibodies will be ready for the allergen the next time.

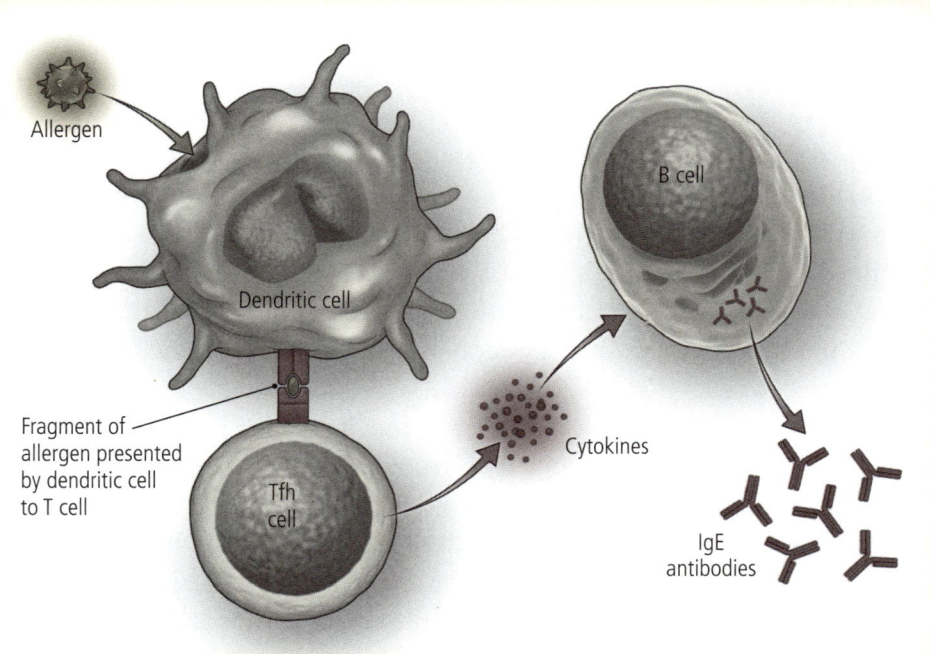

2. Subsequent exposures (allergic reactions): Your IgE antibodies recognize the allergen and trigger an allergic response.

The IgE antibodies that were created on first exposure to the allergen lie in wait on the surface of mast cells, immune system cells found in the mucous membrane layers at the entry points of the body (such as the nose, eyes, lungs, and gut). When an allergen meets up with the IgE antibodies, the mast cell releases pro-inflammatory substances, such as tryptase, histamine, leukotrienes, and prostaglandins, that cause inflammation.

Mast cells also produce their own cytokines that stimulate B cells to produce more IgE, arming more mast cells so that next time the allergen comes along, the reaction is even stronger. At the same time, Th2 cells produce cytokines that stimulate the mast cells, induce their proliferation, and cause local inflammation. Activated mast cells and Th2 cells also recruit other immune cells, known as eosinophils, to the site of the allergic response, increasing local inflammation.

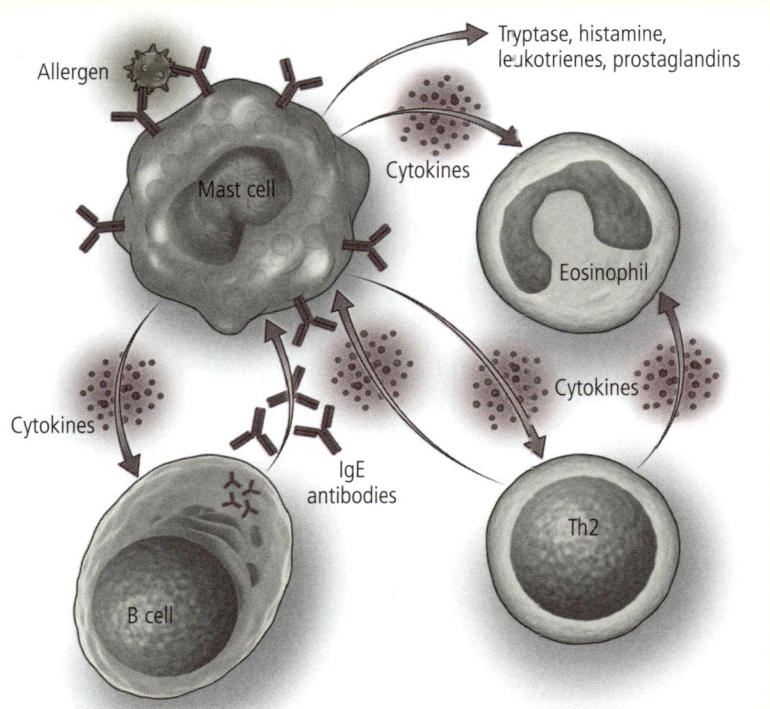

Continued from page 18

with allergic reactions. Many have a personal or family history of other allergic conditions such as asthma, food allergies, and hay fever. Hypersensitivity to substances in the environment, including pollen and pet dander, can trigger flare-ups of eczema, especially in people who have a severe case. However, eczema is not caused by an allergic reaction to substances touching the skin; that's a separate condition called allergic contact dermatitis.

The telltale red, itchy rash is the obvious symptom of eczema, but under the skin's surface, a lot more is going on. The skin manifestation is the result of an abnormal immune reaction that produces inflammation inside the body.

Eczema is sometimes referred to as "the itch that rashes," and for good reason. It starts with an itch, when chemical mediators in the skin stimulate nerve endings in the epidermis. Most people can't help scratching. But when you scratch that itch in an attempt to find relief, more inflammatory substances are released, leading to a repeated sequence of events known as the "itch-scratch cycle."

Every time you scratch your skin, you break down skin cells. Normally, the skin's outer layer, or epidermis, serves as a barrier to prevent allergens, irritants, bacteria, and other unwelcome substances from getting inside. In eczema, this barrier is weaker and more porous than usual, making it more prone to damage and inflammation. Microbes, pet dander, dust mites, and other foreign substances can more easily slip into those damaged areas, compounding the immune reaction. Immune cells near the skin's surface send the alert to Th1 and Th2 cells, which release chemicals that produce the redness and rash. In normal situations, the immune system response would eventually stop. But in eczema it continues, producing a constant state of low-level inflammation. Even when no rash is visible, inflammation persists under the skin.

Asthma

Asthma is a disease of the lungs that involves a complex relationship between allergens and irritants in the environment, overreactive bronchial tubes, and inflammation. Normally when we breathe in, oxygen-saturated air passes into the lungs via two branching tubes known as bronchi, which then branch further into smaller tubes called bronchioles. The inhaled air travels into the grapelike arrangement of small sacs called alveoli at the ends of the bronchioles, where oxygen enters the bloodstream via the network of blood vessels surrounding the alveoli deep in lung tissue.

Asthma used to be understood strictly based on its physical effects on the lungs. Muscles surrounding the bronchial tubes contracted, narrowing these tubes and restricting air flow—or so it was believed. Now, doctors and researchers recognize that asthma is a disease of inflammation that involves the actions of inflammatory cells such as mast cells, eosinophils, and neutrophils, and the release of inflammatory chemicals such as histamine, leukotrienes, and a variety of cytokines. Inflammation, plus constriction of the surrounding muscles, is what causes the narrowing of the bronchial tubes. The narrowing leaves less space for air to flow into the lungs. This constriction of airflow leads to the telltale symptoms of asthma—shortness of breath, wheezing, and chest tightness.

What triggers this inflammatory process is unique to each person. In people with allergic asthma, exposure to typical allergens such as pollen, animal dander, or dust sets the inflammatory process in motion.

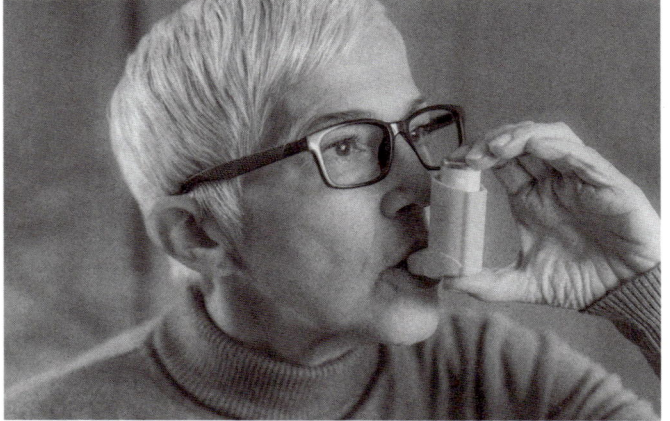
In people with asthma, the airways in the lungs always show some degree of inflammation. But during an attack, the airways swell up, blocking airflow. Medications called bronchodilators can help.

In nonallergic asthma, symptoms are triggered not by allergens, but by irritants such as smoke, or exercise. Viral infections may also cause asthma flare-ups, especially in children.

Yet even when people with asthma are not exposed to offending substances and they seem to be breathing well, low-level inflammation persists in their bronchial tubes (see Figure 6, at right). What causes this constant state of inflammation is not yet clear, but it makes the bronchial tubes hyperresponsive or "twitchy"—that is, prone to spasm in response to allergens or irritants in the air that wouldn't normally cause a problem.

Persistent inflammation produces long-term, structural changes in the airway, which exacerbate the cycle. The airways thicken and scar. Muscle cells enlarge. Cells of the airways release inflammatory chemicals and sticky mucus. Repeatedly activated mast cells release chemicals that attract eosinophils, which in turn cause more inflammation. All of these changes in tandem make the airway walls swell, narrowing the airways even more.

Bringing down inflammation to treat asthma and allergies

There are two fundamental ways to manage asthma, eczema, and allergies. One is to avoid exposure to triggers like pollen or mold (allergy testing can identify your unique triggers). The other is to take medicines that suppress inflammation and its complications by targeting the processes that underlie symptoms. The main drug treatments for allergies, asthma, and eczema work by dampening inflammation either locally or throughout the body.

Antihistamines block the release of histamine, which causes symptoms like itching, a runny nose, sneezing, and hives. Examples include diphenhydramine (Benadryl) and loratadine (Alavert, Claritin). These drugs work by binding to histamine receptors in mast cells. They treat seasonal and indoor allergies, but they are not effective against asthma.

Corticosteroids are manufactured drugs that are designed to mimic the effects of cortisol, a powerful natural anti-inflammatory hormone the adrenal

Figure 6: How asthma restricts breathing

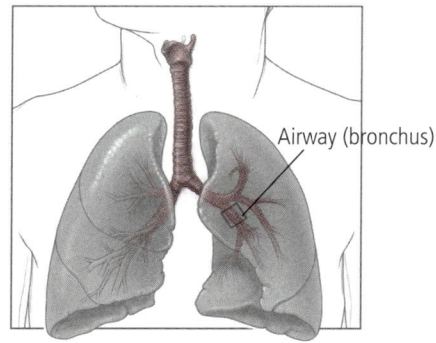

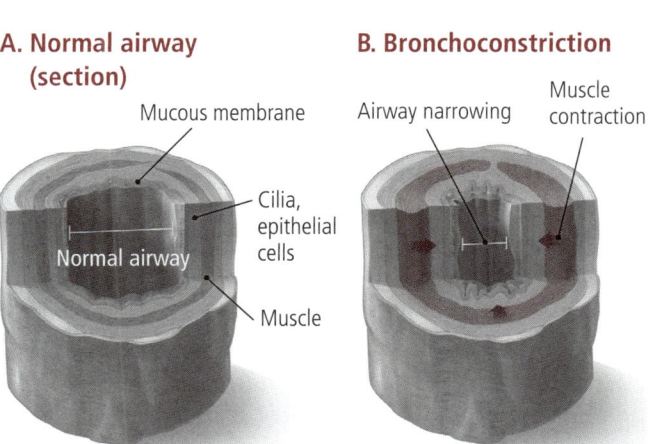

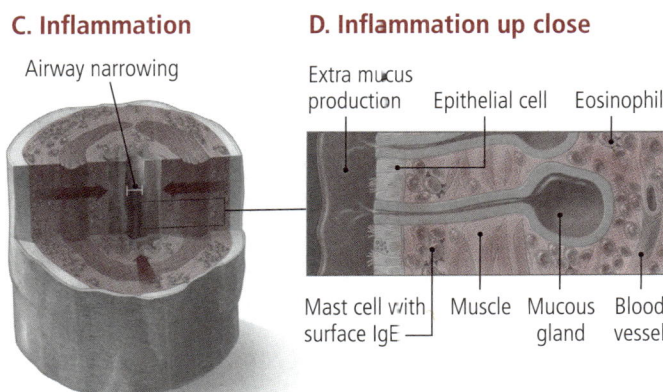

In a normal airway **(A)**, muscles are relaxed so that air easily travels through the airway.

Asthma causes two problems that can restrict breathing. First, the bronchial muscles contract **(B)**, often in response to an allergen or some other asthma trigger. Second, the bronchial walls, which always have some degree of inflammation in people with asthma, become swollen and fill with excess mucus **(C)**. Some of the cells involved in inflammation of the airways are mast cells and eosinophils, which release chemicals that cause the airways to narrow **(D)**.

glands produce. (Corticosteroids are not the same as the anabolic steroids weight lifters sometimes take to increase their strength and muscle mass.) These drugs act directly on inflammatory cells such as mast cells and eosinophils, and they help to reduce cytokine production. When sprayed into the nose, corticosteroid drugs reduce the swelling that causes congestion. When inhaled or taken orally, they suppress the pathways that contribute to airway inflammation and swelling in asthma. Topical steroid creams bring down swelling and relieve itching and rashes in eczema.

Bronchodilators relax tightened muscles around the airways, to allow more air to flow into the lungs. There are three types of bronchodilators: beta-agonists, anticholinergics, and theophylline. These drugs work in one of two ways: short-acting bronchodilators (or "rescue" inhalers) work quickly to stop an asthma attack, while long-acting bronchodilators are taken daily to prevent asthma symptoms.

Leukotriene inhibitors, such as montelukast (Singulair), block the action of leukotrienes, inflammatory chemicals your body releases after it comes in contact with an allergy trigger like mold or pollen. Leukotrienes are what cause symptoms like congestion, a runny nose, and trouble breathing during an allergy or asthma attack.

Immunotherapy—typically in the form of "allergy shots" but sometimes given orally—is another approach to allergies that exposes the body to gradually increasing doses of an allergen. Over a period of weeks or months, the immune system slowly becomes desensitized to the substance. The number of Th2 cells decreases while Th1 cells increase, mast cells and basophils release less of their chemicals upon exposure to the allergen, and B cells produce less IgE. As a result of these effects, allergy symptoms improve.

Immunosuppressant drugs like azathioprine (Azasan, Imuran) and cyclosporine (Neoral) dampen the immune system response to give eczema-afflicted skin a chance to heal. Topical calcineurin inhibitors, such as tacrolimus (Protopic) and pimecrolimus (Elidel), suppress part of the immune response by inhibiting the enzyme calcineurin, which switches on T cells.

Biologics are a newer class of drugs made from living organisms. They are genetically engineered to target specific cells or proteins that control the inflammatory process. Five injectable biologics are FDA-approved to treat asthma in people with severe symptoms that have not responded to other treatments. Omalizumab (Xolair) targets IgE antibodies. Mepolizumab (Nucala), reslizumab (Cinqair), and benralizumab (Fasenra) block interleukin-5 in people with a severe form of asthma. Dupilumab (Dupixent) also treats asthma, and it's the only biologic drug FDA-approved to treat eczema. It blocks two pro-inflammatory cytokines, interleukin-4 and interleukin-13, from binding to their receptors.

A better understanding of the genetic, environmental, and immunologic factors that contribute to allergies and allergic inflammation is helping researchers develop new ways to treat or even prevent allergies—for example, by targeting specific receptors, T cells, cytokines, or other parts of the pathways involved in the allergic inflammatory response. Researchers are also trying to develop more personalized therapies that are allergen-specific or that zero in on an individual's particular allergic response.

Inflammation and autoimmune disease: When your body fights itself

An autoimmune disease is essentially your body's revolt against itself. The immune system, normally tasked with protecting you from external threats, instead directs its assault against healthy tissues and organs. In this case, antibodies (called autoantibodies because they attack your own tissues) and T cells target certain proteins (autoantigens) and launch an immune response against them.

More than 100 different autoimmune diseases exist. Together, they afflict more than 23 million Americans, with women disproportionally affected. Some autoimmune conditions, like multiple sclerosis, rheumatoid arthritis, and type 1 diabetes, are well known. Others, like Behcet's disease, giant cell arteritis, and Goodpasture's syndrome, may be less familiar.

What causes the body to turn against itself? Theories about the origins of autoimmune diseases abound. Genetics undoubtedly play a role. These conditions run in families, and anyone with a parent or sibling who has multiple sclerosis, lupus, or another one of these conditions faces an increased risk. Sometimes the predisposition for autoimmunity, rather than the specific disease, is inherited. For example, someone who has a close relative with rheumatoid arthritis may instead develop lupus.

Genes don't tell the whole story, however. More likely, genes merely set the stage, and then environmental exposures actually set the disease in motion. Exposure to cigarette smoke and pollution have both been implicated in autoimmune diseases such as rheumatoid arthritis. Chemicals in smoke and pollutants may induce cellular damage that produces inflammation and launches the immune response. Some researchers believe that these diseases are the result of collateral damage that occurs when healthy cells get caught up in the immune system charge against an infection.

Below are some of the most common autoimmune diseases, listed alphabetically. While this is not a complete directory, it does offer a snapshot of how autoimmune diseases work, the role that inflammation plays in them, and the way therapies that address inflammation treat them.

Inflammatory bowel disease (IBD)

Inflammatory bowel disease is a broad term that refers to two inflammatory conditions affecting the digestive system: Crohn's disease and ulcerative colitis. Both conditions cause ulcers and inflammation in the lining of the intestinal tract. This inflammation alters gut function in a way that gives rise to symptoms like pain, diarrhea, and intense abdominal cramps. There is much overlap of symptoms between the two conditions, which can make them hard to distinguish. Ulcerative colitis, however, is focused mainly in the colon and rectum, while Crohn's disease can cause sores and inflammation anywhere in the digestive tract, from mouth to anus. Inflammation is also what distinguishes IBD from irritable bowel syndrome (IBS). IBS shares symptoms like diarrhea and abdominal cramps with IBD. The main distinguishing features are that with IBS, inspection of the bowel and biopsy samples reveal no significant inflammation or any other specific abnormality.

Although the exact cause of IBD is unknown, there is a strong genetic factor associated with the disease. People who have a parent or sibling with the condition are 10 to 15 times more likely to develop it than are people without this family history. One theory is that this genetic predisposition sets up an abnormal immune system response to intestinal bacteria, which leads to a state of chronic inflammation (see "The role of the microbiome in inflammatory diseases," page 24). Other environmental factors, including smoking, may also be involved in triggering the disease.

Persistent inflammation can permanently damage the intestine and may raise the risk for colorectal cancer in people with IBD. People with IBD also have a heightened risk of inflammatory eye and skin conditions, as well as for chronic inflammation in their lungs and airways, blood clots, and disorders of the liver and bile ducts.

Lupus

Unlike some autoimmune diseases, which target a specific body part like the joints or skin, systemic lupus erythematosus, or lupus as it is more familiarly known, may affect many parts of the body. It causes inflammation throughout the body, affecting the skin, joints, lungs, heart, kidneys, eyes, digestive system, muscles, and even the brain. The sheer number of organ systems involved leads to a constellation of symptoms—including fatigue, painful joints, fever, anemia, chest pain, butterfly-shaped rash on the face, light sensitivity, mouth sores, and difficulty breathing—which can make diagnosing this disease complex and time-consuming.

As with other diseases that fall under the autoimmune umbrella, lupus's origins are unclear, but it is likely that it similarly stems from a combination of genes and environmental triggers. Researchers have identified more than 50 genes that increase susceptibility to the disease. When one identical twin has lupus, the other one has about a 30% chance of also developing it. Shared genes are probably one reason why certain ethnic groups, including people of African and Asian descent, have a higher prevalence of lupus.

In people who have inherited a genetic susceptibility to lupus, it's possible that something in the environment flips the switch to turn the disease on. What that "switch" might be isn't clear. It might be that an infection (which has not yet been discovered) triggers an abnormal immune response in people who are susceptible to this "misfiring" because of the genetic wiring of their immune system.

One important feature of lupus is an impaired ability to remove old and damaged cells from the body. As cellular debris builds up, it provides a constant source of autoantigens for the immune system to target. Dead cells release substances that continually call in the immune system, which then attacks the body's tissues.

Environmental triggers can also set lupus symptoms in motion. The sun's ultraviolet rays, viral illnesses, certain medications, exhaustion, stress, and injury can all provoke an immune reaction that leads to disease flares.

The role of the microbiome in inflammatory diseases

The human body is more than simply a collection of cells, tissues, and organs. An entire microscopic world, teeming with more than 100 trillion bacteria, fungi, viruses, and protozoa, inhabits your gut and other parts of your body. These microorganisms outnumber your own cells by a factor of 10 to one.

While some members of your microbiome can make you sick, most live harmoniously and even helpfully within you. Beneficial bacteria help your body digest food, produce vitamins, protect you against the harmful bacteria, and inhibit inflammation.

Although the makeup of your microbiome remains fairly stable, certain environmental factors—including a high-calorie, high-fat diet and drugs like antibiotics—can change its composition. Some of these changes can damage the barrier that keeps these bacteria out of the bloodstream. Once the barrier is damaged, bacteria may cause inflammation in the digestive tract and throughout the body (although just how this happens is uncertain). Research has found that an imbalance in the microbiome, called dysbiosis, may contribute to the development of autoimmune diseases like inflammatory bowel disease, rheumatoid arthritis and other inflammatory types of arthritis, type 1 diabetes, multiple sclerosis, and lupus.

Studies are currently investigating whether probiotics (foods and supplements that contain live beneficial bacteria) and prebiotics (foods and supplements that feed and encourage the growth of beneficial bacteria) might help to treat people with autoimmune diseases. So far, this research has been inconclusive. Another promising therapy under investigation is fecal transplantation, which transfers a sample of the microbiome from a healthy donor to a person with autoimmune disease. And still other research is focused on how certain diets—such as the Mediterranean diet—might alter the gut microenvironment in a way that dampens inflammation in autoimmune diseases.

Multiple sclerosis

In multiple sclerosis (MS), the immune system attack is directed against the central nervous system. The body's nerves transmit electrical signals from the brain and spinal cord to the rest of the body and from the body back to the spinal cord and brain. These messages control just about everything you do—picking up a glass of water, jogging, talking on a cellphone. In MS, however, this vital network comes under attack.

The specific target of the attack is the myelin sheath that covers and protects your nerves. Made of protein and fat, this sheath insulates the nerves, much like the rubber or plastic coating on electrical wires in your home. The inflammatory attack on myelin not only damages this protective coating, but also destroys nerve fibers, producing areas of scarring—or sclerosis—in the brain and spinal cord. Nerve damage interrupts normal message transmission, causing a host of symptoms, including walking difficulties, numbness and tingling, muscle spasms, weakness, vision problems, and bladder issues.

Again, genes seem to set up the processes that lead to MS, although researchers have not pinpointed the exact genetic targets just yet. One theory about the disease's origins is that, after an infection with a virus like Epstein-Barr, measles, or herpes, the virus lies dormant in the body for many years, only to eventually reawaken and provoke an inflammatory immune response. A newer school of thought postulates that trauma to the brain from a head injury, particularly during the teenage years, might be behind the autoimmune process. A 2017 study found that people who'd had a concussion between ages 10 and 20 were 20% more likely to have MS than those who'd never had a concussion.

Psoriasis

Although psoriasis manifests as a skin disease, it actually starts deep inside the body, the result of an immune system abnormality that causes inflammation.

When you suffer an injury to the skin, T cells usually heal the injury (see "Act 2: Innate immunity," page 8). But in psoriasis, overactive T cells cause healthy skin cells, called keratinocytes, to multiply much faster than usual. Typically, new cells are made in the lower layers of epidermis (the outermost skin layer). They gradually rise to the surface, and then die off and shed when the body no longer needs them. The process generally takes about four weeks. But in psoriasis, the rapidly multiplying skin cells move to the surface within just four or five days, far too quickly for the body to efficiently dispose of them. The excess skin cells pile up on the surface of the skin, forming inflamed, red, scaly patches known as plaques. T cells also send out distress signals in the form of cytokines—chemicals such as tumor necrosis factor (TNF) and interleukin-2—which produce inflammation in the skin and other organs.

Psoriasis can occur in different places on the body, with slightly different symptoms. The most common form, plaque psoriasis, causes plaques to form on areas like the elbows, knees, and scalp. In about 15% of people with psoriasis, immune cells migrate to joints like the knees, fingers, and toes, and trigger inflammation known as psoriatic arthritis.

Researchers don't know exactly what causes the immune system to go after healthy skin cells in psoriasis, but there is a strong genetic component to the disease. About 40% of people with psoriasis or psoriatic arthritis have a family member with the disorder. Other factors also play a role. Psoriasis usually flares up in response to some inciting environmental event, such as a stressful day at work, an infection like strep throat, a cut or other skin injury, heavy drinking, smoking, or the use of medications like beta blockers (used to treat high blood pressure) or lithium (prescribed for mood disorders).

Rheumatoid arthritis

Inflammation is a key component of all autoimmune joint diseases, including psoriatic arthritis, lupus, and Sjögren's syndrome. Rheumatoid arthritis is the most common of these conditions, afflicting more than 1.3 million Americans. Arthritis in general is characterized by joint inflammation; in the case of rheumatoid arthritis, the disease most often attacks multiple joints and is usually symmetrical, affecting joints on both sides of the body, particularly the finger joints, bases

Figure 7: Joint changes in rheumatoid arthritis

Rheumatoid arthritis can affect all of the structures surrounding a joint.

A. Inflammation begins in the synovium, the lining of an otherwise normal joint.

B. Synovial cells begin to proliferate and form pannus—a rough, grainy tissue that grows into the space between the bones.

C. Cells in the pannus release substances that eat into cartilage and bone, causing bone erosion.

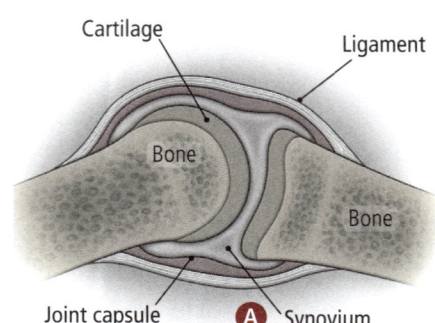
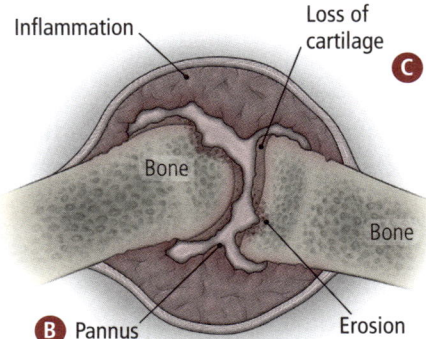

The damage often does not stop there. Nearby tendons and the joint capsule may also become inflamed. All of this damage to joint structures can cause pain, instability, deformity, weakness, loss of motion, and, occasionally, rupture of tendons.

Rheumatoid arthritis and heart disease

People with rheumatoid arthritis face double the usual odds of developing heart disease, a threat that is not entirely attributable to typical risk factors like high blood pressure, diabetes, high cholesterol, or smoking. Experts say the connection more likely stems from inflammation. The same inflammatory processes that target the synovium in joints can also harm the heart (see "Inflammation and your heart," page 38). Inflammation damages blood vessel linings and allows the buildup of fatty deposits called plaques, which narrow arteries, raise blood pressure, and increase the risk for a heart attack or stroke. Hardening of the arteries (atherosclerosis) not only is more common in people with rheumatoid arthritis than in the general population, but also progresses at a faster rate.

The good news is that controlling joint inflammation in rheumatoid arthritis appears to protect the heart, too. Some of the medications used to treat rheumatoid arthritis, including methotrexate, have been shown to prevent cardiovascular disease progression and lower the risk of dying from heart disease.

Other drugs may be more problematic for people with rheumatoid arthritis. Nonsteroidal anti-inflammatory drugs, used to control pain and swelling in arthritis, can raise blood pressure, and they have been linked to a higher risk of heart attack and stroke. Whether it's safe for you to take these drugs may depend in part on your existing heart risk factors. If you have high blood pressure, cholesterol, or other heart disease risk factors, talk to your doctor about whether you may want to look elsewhere for pain relief.

of the thumbs, wrists, elbows, knees, ankles, or feet.

In rheumatoid arthritis, a faulty immune response initiates the inflammation, which begins in the tissue lining the joints (the synovium; see Figure 7, above). Synovial and other cells produce chemicals, including cytokines, that destroy joints from the inside. The process that leads to joint inflammation may begin long before the symptoms of stiffness, pain, and swelling become apparent. Five years or more before joints show any signs of inflammation, researchers have detected autoantibodies, as well as inflammatory cytokines, in the blood of people who later develop rheumatoid arthritis.

Ongoing inflammation ultimately damages nearby tissues, including bone, tendons, ligaments, and cartilage (the cushioning material within joints). The cells of the synovial tissue also begin to multiply, causing the normally smooth synovium to form a rough, grainy tissue (pannus) that grows into the joint cavity and erodes cartilage. If the tendons become inflamed, they may shorten and immobilize the joint. If the tendons rupture, the joint may become loose or floppy.

Over time, the ligaments and tendons that hold bones in place can also stretch and weaken, causing bones to become misaligned. Making an accurate diagnosis of rheumatoid arthritis, as early as possible, is crucial to reduce disability. Without the proper treatment, inflammation can permanently damage the affected joints.

Rheumatoid arthritis is a progressive systemic disease, meaning that over time it may affect many targets or even the body as a whole. In addition to the joints, inflammation can affect the skin, eyes, lungs, and blood vessels. Other complications include lung, heart, and neurologic disorders. For example, lung scarring (pulmonary fibrosis), inflammation of the heart lining (pericarditis), and carpal tunnel syndrome (pain and numbness in the hands and fingers caused by compression of a nerve in the wrist) are well-known complications of rheumatoid arthritis (see "Rheumatoid arthritis and heart disease," page 26).

Type 1 diabetes

Both type 1 and type 2 diabetes are a result of the body's inability to properly move glucose (sugar) from the bloodstream into the cells. The difference between the two conditions is that type 1 diabetes is autoimmune in nature and is marked by insufficient production of insulin by the pancreas, while type 2 diabetes is not considered autoimmune and develops because cells throughout the body become resistant to the effects of insulin, so that the pancreas eventually fails to keep up with the increased demand. Type 1 diabetes used to be known as "juvenile diabetes" to distinguish it from type 2 diabetes, which generally struck in older adulthood. But with the increase in type 2 diabetes among young adults and even teens and children, the term has fallen out of use.

In people with type 1 diabetes, the immune system attacks insulin-producing beta cells in the pancreas. Normally, healthy beta cells release insulin in response to rising blood sugar, as carbohydrates from food are broken down into glucose. Insulin attaches to cells like a key, essentially unlocking them so that they can absorb sugar to use for energy. Insulin then directs any leftover sugar to the liver, where it is stored and can be released when supplies run low.

In type 1 diabetes, however, damage from the autoimmune attack prevents beta cells from producing and releasing insulin. When more than 90% of the beta cells have been destroyed, symptoms of high blood sugar, including extreme thirst and excess urination, appear. High blood sugar damages blood vessels throughout the body. It also acts as a warning call to the immune system, which produces chronic inflammation in response. The combination of inflammation and high blood sugar eventually damages organs like the kidneys, heart, and eyes, as well as nerves and blood vessels. People with type 1 diabetes need to take insulin for the rest of their lives to control their blood sugar.

Like other autoimmune diseases, type 1 diabetes has both environmental and genetic causes. If both parents have type 1 diabetes, their child may have a risk as high as 25% of developing the disease. That's 75 times higher than the risk among members of the general population. But among identical twins, if one twin has the disease, the risk of the other one developing it is higher still—50% by age 40.

One theory is that in people who are genetically susceptible, an environmental trigger sets off the immune response. One possible trigger is a virus like mumps, rubella, enterovirus, or coxsackievirus. In one study, genetically susceptible children who had respiratory infections in their first year of life were more

> ### Is osteoarthritis an inflammatory disease?
>
> Osteoarthritis is by far the most common form of arthritis, affecting more than 30 million people in the United States alone. It is marked by gradual damage to articular cartilage, the type that lines the ends of bones in joints like the knees, shoulders, elbows, and wrists. Osteoarthritis was once thought to be a solely mechanical and degenerative process, stemming from the gradual wearing-away of protective cartilage in the joints from years of running, jumping, and other activities. That origin story earned it the nickname "wear and tear" arthritis.
>
> In recent years, researchers have begun to look at this disease in a new light. Studies have revealed the presence of inflammatory cells like T cells in synovial tissue (the membrane that lines a joint's inner surface). While the numbers of these cells are not as high as they are in autoimmune forms of arthritis, they are significant enough for the medical community to consider osteoarthritis a disease at least in part related to inflammation. Given the low-grade chronic inflammation that appears to exist in osteoarthritis, doctors are considering whether biologic drugs like the ones currently used to treat rheumatoid arthritis might one day have an application in treating chronic osteoarthritis as well.

likely to develop type 1 diabetes. Exposure to toxins may also help set in motion the autoimmune cascade of events. Experts believe that as the immune system attempts to rid the body of the virus or toxin, it mistakenly destroys beta cells in the process.

The hallmark of type 1 diabetes is inflammation of the pancreatic islets—the tissue that contains insulin-producing beta cells. This inflammation is known as insulitis. It appears that multiple immune cell types converge to bring about the destruction of beta cells. Researchers have discovered an abundant supply of lymphocytes, neutrophils, and natural killer T cells in and around the islets.

If inflammation is at play in type 1 diabetes, then it would make a logical treatment target. Studies have investigated a number of possible immunotherapeutic treatments that focus on the inflammatory process, such as the monoclonal antibody rituximab (Rituxan). So far, these investigations have produced only minimal success, in part because studies have only included people whose beta cells have already suffered a significant amount of immune-induced damage. Researchers say the only way to achieve a true cure for type 1 diabetes with immunotherapy would be to treat people before there has been extensive damage or to somehow replace those beta cells that have been lost.

Taming inflammation to treat autoimmune diseases

Treatment for most autoimmune diseases today involves the use of drugs that bring down inflammation or suppress the immune response.

Nonsteroidal anti-inflammatory drugs (NSAIDs) like aspirin, ibuprofen (Advil, Motrin), and naproxen (Naprosyn, Aleve) have both pain-relieving and anti-inflammatory effects. They work by blocking cyclo-oxygenase (COX) enzymes. These enzymes promote the production of prostaglandins—hormones that form from chemical reactions at the site of an injury or infection. While prostaglandins promote healing, they also cause inflammation and pain. Blocking COX enzymes inhibits these effects. But these drugs can also cause gastric bleeding and stomach ulcers, and they have been linked to heart problems, including heart attacks and heart failure.

Corticosteroids like prednisone regulate the production of cytokines and other inflammatory substances, to bring down inflammation in affected areas of the gut, joints, skin, or elsewhere. Doctors first used these drugs in the 1940s to reduce joint swelling and ease pain in people with rheumatoid arthritis, and they are now used to treat a number of inflammatory diseases, including asthma. Their effectiveness comes at a cost, however—severe side effects like infection, weight gain, and bone thinning. Therefore, corticosteroids are often prescribed for short-term use only. They can bring down inflammation and ease pain temporarily, but they are generally incapable of slowing the onward progression of autoimmune diseases.

Conventional immunosuppressive drugs—including methotrexate, azathioprine (Imuran, Azasan), and cyclophosphamide (Cytoxan, Neosar)—can actually slow and sometimes even halt the damage inflicted by the immune system on joints, skin, nerves, and other tissues, particularly when started early in the course of the disease. These immunosuppressive medications inhibit the production of cytokines and other inflammatory substances to suppress the impact of the immune response. However, they must be used with caution, because calming the immune system also reduces its ability to fight infections.

Biologic drugs are a newer form of immunosuppressants, derived from living cells or containing components of living organisms. Monoclonal antibodies and other types of biologic drugs target specific proteins that contribute to the immune response and lead to inflammation. For example, TNF inhibitors like adalimumab (Humira), etanercept (Enbrel), and infliximab (Remicade) block TNF, a cytokine that plays a major role in the immune and inflammatory responses. Biologics that target other pro-inflammatory cytokines have also been developed. For example, tocilizumab (Actemra) blocks IL-6 to treat people with rheumatoid arthritis who haven't improved enough while on anti-TNF therapy. Because biologic drugs are more selective about what they attack than older immunosuppressants, they also produce fewer side effects. However, they have been linked to an increased risk for infections like tuberculosis and pneumonia. ▼

SPECIAL SECTION

Combating chronic inflammation with lifestyle changes

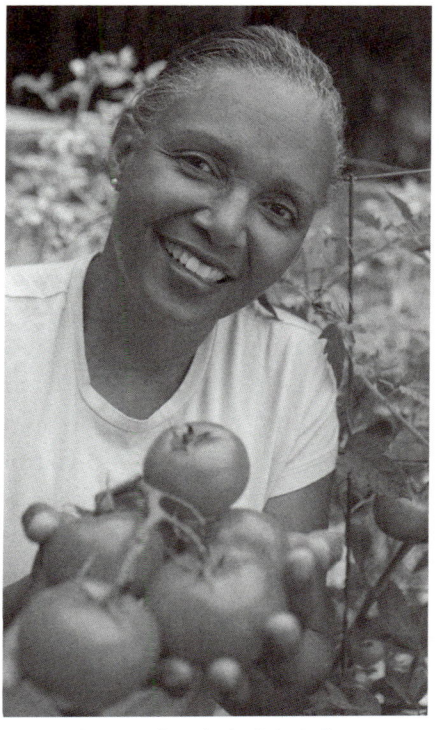

Diets rich in produce help fight inflammation. Despite persistent claims, there is no evidence that foods from the nightshade family (like tomatoes) promote inflammation.

As this report has explained so far, there are many obvious causes of inflammation, ranging from wounds and viruses to allergies and autoimmune diseases. But there are also many subtler causes of inflammation—including obesity, an unhealthy diet, smoking, alcohol use, chronic sleep deprivation, and a sedentary lifestyle—that may be the result of choices we make every day. Over the years, this ongoing, low-grade inflammation can contribute to the development of major medical conditions like heart disease, type 2 diabetes, certain cancers, and even depression, all of which are discussed in later chapters.

This Special Section focuses on the strategies you can use to help combat this chronic inflammation and its many insidious effects. That's not to say that adopting this program is an ironclad guarantee against developing these diseases—or that you can manage these conditions with lifestyle changes alone once you have them—but such changes can definitely help. Below are some of the best-researched strategies for taming inflammation that is lifestyle-related.

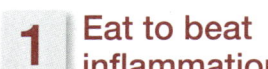

1 Eat to beat inflammation

Your diet plays an important role in setting off chronic inflammation. One reason lies deep inside your gut. Digestive bacteria release chemicals that may spur or suppress inflammation. The types of bacteria that populate your gut and their chemical byproducts vary according to the foods you eat. Some foods encourage the growth of bacteria that stimulate inflammation, while others promote the growth of bacteria that suppress it (see "How diet can transform the microbiome," page 30). Another reason for the connection is obesity. Eating too much—especially the wrong types of foods—leads to weight gain, which is itself a cause of inflammation. Some foods trigger inflammation independently of their ability to promote weight gain, suggesting that some diets are more pro-inflammatory than others.

Inflammation is a big buzzword in health and nutrition—for

good reason, considering the number of health conditions linked to chronic, systemic inflammation. That said, where there's buzz, there's hype, and many "anti-inflammatory" diets touted in books and online are not grounded in science.

When considering any diet that claims it will end inflammation, be wary. The science to back up these claims is generally slim or nonexistent. Epidemiological studies, which look at rates of disease in populations, do find that people who eat diets high in certain foods—fruits, vegetables, whole grains, fatty fish, nuts, and healthy oils (essentially the Mediterranean diet)—have lower rates of chronic conditions such as heart disease and cancer. What these studies can't prove is whether these lower rates of disease are directly attributable to the foods participants ate, or to other factors, such as more exercise.

Certain foods have been spotlighted in the media for their supposed ability to fight inflammation—among them ginger, onions, turmeric, and berries. Yet researchers don't know how much of these each of these foods we would need to eat to see a specific benefit. In any case, the levels of antioxidant and anti-inflammatory compounds in agricultural products vary according to growing conditions (such as weather and soil quality) and storage conditions (such as temperature and shelf time), so there is no way to standardize a dietary prescription as pharmaceutical companies standardize drugs.

To practice "anti-inflammatory eating," it's best to focus on an overall healthy diet (see "The best anti-inflammatory diets," page 31). The same diet that protects your heart and keeps your weight in check also tends to bring down inflammation. That means one that emphasizes fruits, vegetables, nuts, whole grains, fish, and healthy oils, and limits food loaded with simple sugars (like soda and candy), beverages that contain high-fructose corn syrup (like juice drinks and sports drinks), and refined carbohydrates.

Vegetables. Most brightly colored vegetables naturally contain high levels of protective compounds. Green, leafy vegetables like spinach, kale, collard greens, and broccoli contain antioxidants that protect cells from the damaging effects of free radicals. Onions are a rich source of anti-inflammatory polyphenols. Lycopene, a nutrient in tomatoes, may help reduce the inflammation that contributes to cancer growth and spread.

Fruits. The same chemicals that give berries and other fruits their brilliant hues also imbue them with nutrients. When choosing fruits, the more color in your basket, the better. Berries, including strawberries, blueberries, and raspberries, are an especially rich source of antioxidants and anti-inflammatory chemicals. Eat them on their own, or use them to top salads, oatmeal, and frozen yogurt. Grapes, plums, and cherries are abundant sources of polyphenols, and they have been shown in animal studies to reduce cytokine production.

Nuts and seeds. Nuts are nutritional powerhouses. They provide protein, fiber, antioxidants,

> ### How diet can transform the microbiome
>
> You can see the effects of a healthy diet pretty easily in the forms of weight loss and energy gain. When you eat anti-inflammatory foods, a lot happens under the surface, too. Not only do markers of inflammation in your blood drop, but your gut also undergoes a real and dramatic population shift.
>
> The gut microbiota (the bacteria and other microorganisms that inhabit your digestive tract) include both beneficial bacteria that aid in processes like digestion and nutrient absorption, and harmful bacteria that contribute to inflammation, illness, and metabolic dysfunction. When it comes to these tiny residents, diversity is an asset. People with a more diverse population of bacteria in their digestive tract tend to have less chronic, low-grade inflammation than those with less diversity. Certain styles of eating—such as a low-sugar, low-fat, high-fiber diet—promote a wider variety of microorganisms in your gut. Probiotics, consumed either as foods (sauerkraut, kimchi, kefir, miso) or supplements, contain beneficial bacteria themselves. Other foods, called prebiotics (which contain fermentable fibers that bacteria like to feed on), are found in foods like onions, bananas, leeks, garlic, oats, and soybeans.

and unsaturated fats that help lower cholesterol and protect your heart. Some varieties of nuts and seeds are also high in alpha-linolenic acid, a type of omega-3 fatty acid with anti-inflammatory properties. Studies have found that consuming nuts and seeds is associated with reduced markers of inflammation and a lower risk of cardiovascular disease and type 2 diabetes. In one study, people who replaced three servings of meat, eggs, or refined grains a week with the same number of nut servings had significantly lower measures of systemic inflammation in their blood.

Fatty fish. Fatty fish such as salmon, sardines, anchovies, and mackerel offer healthy doses of the omega-3 fatty acids eicosapentaenoic acid and docosahexaenoic acid, which have long been known to reduce inflammation. The power of omega-3s in combating inflammation lies in their ability to disrupt cytokine production, which is key to the body's inflammatory response. Because omega-3s can cross the blood-brain barrier, they may even help lower inflammation associated with Alzheimer's disease and reduce the risk of stroke. Your body can't make these fatty acids, so you need to get them from foods. If you're not a fan of fish, you might try an omega-3 supplement, although there is no solid evidence that taking omega-3s in pill form can lower your risk for heart disease, cancer, or other diseases linked to inflammation.

The best anti-inflammatory diets

When it comes to fighting inflammation with diet, following a specific program is not a necessity. In fact, many of the so-called anti-inflammatory diets are more hype than real science. That said, a couple of diets round up all the anti-inflammatory elements into one eating plan and have more evidence of benefit than other diets. If you aren't sure where to start, these diets are good choices.

Mediterranean diet. People who live in countries ringing the Mediterranean Sea, like Italy and Greece, have traditionally eaten a diet consisting mainly of fruits and vegetables, nuts and seeds, whole grains, fish, and olive oil—the same foods that experts recommend to bring down inflammation. Over the years, researchers began to discover that people who followed this style of eating had lower rates of disease and lived longer than people in the United States who ate a Western-style diet.

The Mediterranean diet is ranked high among doctors and dietitians, and for good reason. Studies show it protects against diseases linked to inflammation, including cardiovascular disease, metabolic syndrome, and type 2 diabetes. And, because it includes a variety of foods, the Mediterranean diet is relatively easy to follow and stick with.

DASH diet. Although its name may suggest the "grab-and-go" section of the supermarket, DASH is anything but a fast-food regimen. DASH stands for Dietary Approaches to Stop Hypertension. It was originally developed to lower blood pressure without medication, but is now widely considered to be one of the healthiest eating patterns around. It includes foods low in total fat, saturated fat, and cholesterol, and lots of fruits, vegetables, and whole grains. Protein is supplied by low-fat dairy, fish, poultry, and nuts. Red meat, sweets, and sugary drinks are limited. DASH is high in fiber, potassium, calcium, and magnesium and low in sodium.

Dr. Andrew Weil's Anti-Inflammatory Diet. Another anti-inflammatory diet with science to back it up comes from Harvard-educated integrative medicine practitioner Dr. Andrew Weil. He started talking up anti-inflammatory measures decades ago, long before the idea began trending. His anti-inflammatory diet could be described as a Mediterranean diet with Asian influences. About 40% to 50% of calories come from carbohydrates, 30% from fat, and 20% to 30% from protein.

Where Dr. Weil's diet wins is in its emphasis on plant-based foods and healthy protein sources, as well as specific elements (fatty fish, fruits, vegetables, oils, nuts, and seeds) that help to reduce inflammation. It also minimizes highly processed foods, which can contribute to inflammation.

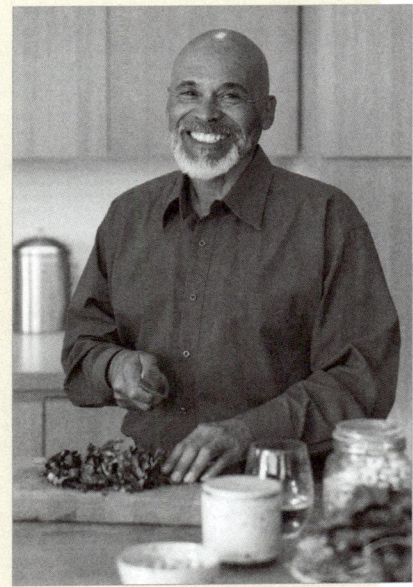

One common feature of all good anti-inflammatory diets is a hefty dose of produce. Healthful oils like olive oil also help.

Healthy oils. Oils are another abundant source of unsaturated fatty acids, provided you choose them wisely. The best anti-inflammatory oils are olive oil, walnut oil, flaxseed oil, and canola oil, which may help lower cholesterol and heart disease risk. Use them in cooking and drizzle them on salads.

Beverages. What you drink can also influence levels of inflammation in your body. Coffee contains polyphenols and other anti-inflammatory compounds. It's a healthy drink, provided you don't load it up with cream and sugar. Green tea is also rich in both polyphenols and antioxidants.

Not surprisingly, foods that contribute to inflammation are the same ones that are generally considered bad for other aspects of health. These include sodas and refined carbohydrates (like white bread, sugar-filled lattes, and cake), as well as red meat and processed meats (hot dogs, bologna). Such unhealthy foods are also likely to contribute to weight gain, which is itself a risk factor for inflammation. In addition, certain components or ingredients in processed foods, like the emulsifiers added to ice cream, may have effects on inflammation.

2 Exercise regularly

The government and most major health organizations urge us all to get at least 150 minutes (two-and-a-half hours) of aerobic activity plus two or three strength training sessions every week. A solid body of research shows that regular exercise helps to protect the heart and brain, strengthen the bones, and prevent diseases like dementia, type 2 diabetes, heart disease, and depression. It may even lengthen your life.

Exercise causes many changes in the body that produce these positive effects. But one important factor that is often underappreciated is that it helps fight low-grade chronic inflammation—the same type of inflammation that underlies so many chronic diseases.

The research into exercise and inflammation is still young, but it has already yielded fascinating insights. For example, regular exercise seems to control inflammation in multiple ways. By helping to prevent excess weight gain, it indirectly heads off the proliferation of inflammation-promoting macrophages in fat tissue. It can also have more direct effects on levels of pro-inflammatory cytokines. For example, in a study by researchers at the University of California San Diego, published in 2017 in *Brain, Behavior and Immunity*, just 20 minutes of moderate aerobic exercise lowered production of TNF. The authors noted that the anti-inflammatory effect may come from catecholamines, hormones the adrenal glands release during exercise.

The caveat is that if you overdo it—say, by exercising at too high an intensity or for too long—an exercise session can damage muscles and connective tissue and *provoke* an inflammatory response. Before starting or ramping up an exercise program, you should speak with your doctor, especially if you've undergone surgery recently, have musculoskeletal problems, or have a major disease like heart disease. If you work out on a regular basis and know your limits, however, the effects should be overwhelmingly beneficial.

Exercise of all types is good. The point is that you need to do it regularly and observe basic precautions to avoid injury. (Harvard Health Publishing has a number of Special Health Reports on exercise. For more information, see "Resources," page 52.)

Exercise of all types is good for your health. Any amount helps, even if you can't do the recommended amount. More is better than some. Some is better than none.

3 Manage your weight

Excess weight is a known contributor to inflammation. Scientists now realize that body fat is more than just inert bulk your body carries around. Rather, fat tissue actively produces a wide variety of hormones and pro-inflammatory chemicals (see "Inflammation and metabolic disease," page 46).

This effect helps explain the consistent role obesity plays in heart disease, diabetes, and other metabolically linked chronic diseases. Abdominal fat in particular seems important as a risk factor for cardiovascular disease. Not surprisingly, maintaining a body mass index in the normal range significantly reduces the risk of cardiovascular disease, diabetes, and other conditions that may cause or contribute to inflammation.

Although diet and exercise are frequently cited as the path to weight loss, diet is the more powerful of the two when it comes to shedding pounds—in part, because exercise tends to make you eat more to replace calories you've burned off.

A formal diet is one approach, but simply limiting your portion sizes can also help. One trick is to dish out food in the kitchen, rather than placing serving dishes on the table, where you're tempted to ladle more onto your plate. Try not to nibble when clearing the dishes. And try "closing the kitchen" after a certain hour at night, so you don't go in and snack, particularly

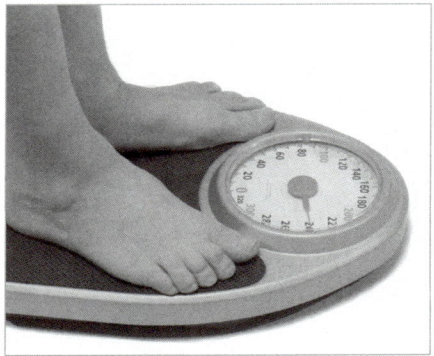

Managing your weight is an important part of fighting inflammation. Fat cells produce a variety of pro-inflammatory chemicals, which play a role in diseases like diabetes.

if late-night snacking is a problem for you.

Another helpful tool is keeping a food diary, so you become aware of how much you're actually eating. Write down everything—those crackers you ate as a midmorning snack, those few squares of chocolate. You might be surprised to find out how much you're consuming since much of it is consumed almost mindlessly while doing other things. When you start paying attention to how much you're eating, you become more careful about caloric intake.

One of the most reliable ways to reduce calories in a healthful way is to increase your intake of vegetables, which are densely packed with nutrients and fiber, but are low in calories. At the same time, it's important to reduce added sugars (sugar that is added in cooking or manufacturing). Many people have particular difficulty reducing added sugars. Here are some tips to help you do that:

Give your brain time to adapt. If you normally drink three cans of soda a day, eliminate one can and replace it with a sugar-free beverage such as flavored seltzer. Eventually you'll want to cut out all three.

Use sweet-tasting herbs and spices. While many herbs and spices are savory, others—including mint, cinnamon, allspice, clove, and nutmeg—add a touch of sweetness to your food. Try substituting cinnamon for sugar in your coffee or oatmeal, or use mint to sweeten your iced tea or even yogurt.

Rely on fruit for dessert. Apples and oranges are naturally sweet. Add a little cream to your berries to make them seem like a special treat. Or try sautéed banana slices; when they come off the stove, add a squeeze of lemon, and top them with pecans or cashews. These options are much more flavorful than most donuts, ice cream, and other sugary desserts.

Drink sweet-tasting teas. Many herbal teas have enough natural sweetness to satisfy your longing. Look for blends containing sweet-tasting herbs like anise hyssop or mint. Blends containing licorice root are especially sweet, though people with high blood pressure should not drink them too often, because licorice can nudge blood pressure up.

Switch to plain. Whatever flavored food you buy, the added flavor often means added sugar. If fruit-flavored yogurt is your No. 1 added sugar source, replace it with plain yogurt, and add fresh fruit or stevia (a calorie-free herbal sweetener). Instead of a salted caramel mocha Frappuccino (69 grams of sugar at Starbucks), try a regular cappuccino, with just espresso, frothed milk, and cinnamon.

Make your own. You can cook a delicious tomato sauce with zero added sugar, if you start with ripe, flavorful tomatoes. Heirloom varieties, in particular, tend to be especially tasty. And if you make your own, you'll avoid not only added sugar but also preservatives and other additives. Or, if you like to bake, experiment with cutting back on the amount of sugar that recipes call for. With most recipes you can cut 10% of the sugar without ruining the dish. (That's 5 teaspoons for each cup.) With some desserts, especially baked goods that contain sweet fruit (such as an apple or berry crisp), you can cut up to 25%, or sometimes more.

4 Get enough sleep

Up to 70 million Americans are chronically sleep-deprived. The lack of sleep has reached epidemic proportions, according to the CDC. Sleep deprivation is a consequence of our faster-paced and technology-dependent lifestyles. The combination of work stress and the blue-lit technology (cellphones, computers, and tablets) we bring with us into

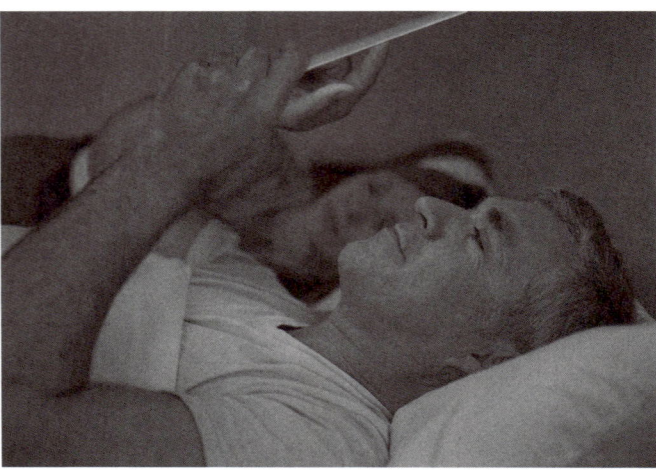

Sleep deprivation—a consequence of our technology-dependent lives—increases inflammation. When the circadian rhythm gets out of whack because of lack of sleep, immune function is affected.

the bedroom prevents us from getting enough restful slumber. For 50 million Americans, the primary sleep disrupter is a disorder like chronic insomnia, sleep apnea, or restless legs syndrome.

Studies have shown that lost sleep produces changes to inflammatory cytokines and other markers of inflammation. When the circadian rhythm gets out of whack because we are not sleeping enough, immune function (along with the rest of the body) is affected too.

Anyone who has spent the overnight hours desperately trying to sleep knows the grogginess and grumpiness the next day can bring. Yet the hazards of poor sleep go far beyond a cranky mood and dampened productivity. Getting fewer than the recommended hours of sleep nightly has also been linked to a higher risk for cardiovascular disease, high blood pressure, diabetes, weight gain, and memory issues. Inadequate sleep—less than seven hours per night—appears to be especially hazardous to heart health. Part of the reason for these health risks is a rise in blood levels of inflammatory substances in poor sleepers. Even a single night of insufficient sleep is enough to disturb your system and spark inflammation, which underscores the need to get into a good sleep routine.

Regularly skimping on sleep also contributes to obesity, which itself is linked with inflammation. With insufficient sleep, you produce higher levels of hunger hormones and lower levels of satiety hormones, causing you to overeat—in particular, you're likely to crave refined carbohydrates. It is also possible that fatigue may cause you to be less physically active, and thus miss out on exercise's weight-loss and anti-inflammatory benefits.

Interestingly, people who sleep too long (beyond nine hours per night) also have high levels of inflammatory substances in their blood. Experts say the ideal sleep time lies somewhere between seven and nine hours nightly. One way to land in that sweet spot is to get your body into the habit by going to bed at the same time every night and waking up seven to nine hours later—the same time every morning. Keep your room quiet, cool, and dark—the optimal conditions for sleep. And leave your devices in another room so you won't be tempted to reach for them in the middle of the night. Instead of indulging in screen time, do something that will wind you down before bed, like reading a book or taking a warm bath.

Managing stress is another crucial element of better sleep. Worries over all the pressures you're under can mount all day and peak right before bedtime, preventing you from getting a restful night. Poor sleep ratchets up the emotional and physical effects of stress, making it even harder to sleep the next night. The stressful day–restless night cycle continues until you can get your stress under control (see "Reduce chronic stress," at right). And stress itself is a trigger for inflammation.

5 Don't smoke

The idea that smoking is bad for your health is by now old news. Tobacco smoke is linked to a veritable medical encyclopedia's worth of diseases, including asthma, multiple types of cancer, chronic obstructive pulmonary disease, diabetes, gum disease, heart disease, and vision loss (from cataracts, macular degeneration, glaucoma, or diabetic retinopathy). Smoking damages blood vessels in a way that makes them more vulnerable to atherosclerosis and resulting cardiovascular disease.

In addition to directly affecting the development of these diseases, smoking also increases your risk for them by promoting inflammation. Smokers have high levels of inflammation, as measured by elevated blood levels of CRP, TNF, and IL-6 (proteins that reflect bodywide inflammation). Smoking also worsens chronic inflammatory diseases such as rheumatoid arthritis and multiple sclerosis. Quitting smoking is good all-around health advice, but it also produces a dramatic drop in inflammatory markers quickly—within just a few weeks.

If you've struggled to kick the habit and failed, don't give up. Many former smokers had to make several attempts and try several cessation methods before finding the one that finally ended their urge to light up. See your doctor for advice on medication and nicotine replacement products to help curb your cravings. Get rid of anything that triggers the desire to smoke—including cigarettes, lighters, and ashtrays. And avoid going to places where you used to light up. If you can't give up smoking on your own, call 800-QUIT-NOW to get advice from trained coaches, or join a support group in your area.

6 Limit alcohol use

When it comes to inflammation, alcohol can be either friend or foe, depending on how you use it. You may have read that moderate alcohol use (one drink daily for women, and one to two drinks for men) reduces the risk of developing diseases linked to inflammation, like heart disease and arthritis. A daily glass of wine does appear to lower markers of inflammation, including CRP, IL-6, and TNF.

Yet the key word is "moderation." Drinking in excess can have the opposite effect, altering the immune system in a way that stimulates the production of pro-inflammatory cytokines. Heavy drinking has been linked to many of the same diseases inflammation promotes, including high blood pressure, stroke, cancer, and dementia.

7 Reduce chronic stress

When our ancestors spotted a spear-wielding foe or a hungry predator, their bodies automatically pumped out hormones like adrenaline, noradrenaline, and cortisol that enabled them to either confront the enemy or run away as quickly as possible. This "fight or flight" response is excellent at protecting us from short-term threats. But when it fires day after day in response to pressures at work or home, it becomes counterproductive and harmful. Such ongoing stress has links to both the development and flare-ups of several chronic inflammatory conditions, including rheumatoid arthritis, cardiovascular disease, depression, and inflammatory bowel disease.

People who engage in regular

SPECIAL SECTION | Combating chronic inflammation with lifestyle changes

relaxation-promoting activities see results not only in the form of lower stress, but also in reduced inflammatory markers. For example, people who regularly practice meditation have lower levels of cortisol and less perceived stress compared with those who don't practice (see "How to lower stress with meditation," below). Regular yoga practice is also associated with lower cortisol levels as well as reduced markers of inflammation.

Meditation and yoga are two common stress-reduction techniques, but there are many other options, which you can choose from based on your personal preferences.

Take a walk outside in a park or forest. Spending time in green spaces has a calming and restorative effect on the mind.

Escape your day. Close your eyes and picture yourself on a beach. Feel the warm sand between your toes. Hear the water gently lapping against the shore. Smell the rich, salty air. Letting your mind wander to a soothing locale, a technique known as creative visualization, can give you a temporary vacation from your worries.

Relax your muscles. Progressive muscle relaxation is a way to let go of any stress you have stored in your muscles. It can also help you fall asleep. Starting at your toes, tense and release one muscle group at a time, working your way up your body. By the time you reach your head, you should have entered a state of total relaxation.

Practice tai chi. This gently flowing exercise program couples slow, purposeful movements with deep breaths. Because tai chi is easy on joints, it is safe for people of all ages and ability levels. And when practiced regularly, it can both reduce stress and improve sleep quality.

Let it out. Before you go to bed, write down everything that has been troubling you in a journal. Releasing your worries through your words is a good way to clear your mind so that you can focus on falling asleep.

Hang out with a friend. Simply spending time with someone who understands you can take a load off your mind. If you use that time to watch a funny movie, you will enjoy the additional benefit of a good laugh on relieving stress.

How to get started on an anti-inflammatory routine

As with any habit or healthy routine, combating inflammation is best started early in life. The sooner you adopt a predominantly plant-based diet, incorporate exercise into your daily routine, get a

How to lower stress with meditation

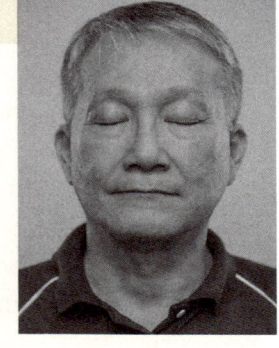

One of the simplest and most effective ways to manage stress is by practicing meditation. It takes just a few minutes, requires no equipment, and can be done anywhere. There are many different types of meditation. Some, like yoga and tai chi, combine movement with deep breathing and mental focus. In one of the most basic techniques, called mindfulness meditation, you focus on your breath and stay rooted in the present moment, pushing any worries out of your mind.

To practice mindfulness meditation:

1. Set aside five or 10 minutes when you know you won't be disturbed. You can set a kitchen timer or an alarm on your smartphone to mark the time.
2. Find a quiet place where there aren't any distractions.
3. Sit on a chair or on a cushion on the floor.
4. Let your gaze gently rest downward, and place your hands on top of your legs.
5. Begin to focus on the sensation of your breath gently moving in and out of your nose or mouth. Feel your chest rise and fall with each breath.
6. Keep your mind focused on the present moment. If it begins to wander, gently steer it back to the present. Think of your worries as clouds. Watch them drift by, rather than dwelling on them.
7. When you are ready to complete your practice, gently bring your attention back into the room. Notice how your body feels in the moment, and what thoughts are going through your mind.

Try to practice mindfulness meditation at least once a day—more often, if you have time.

Build friendships, fight inflammation?

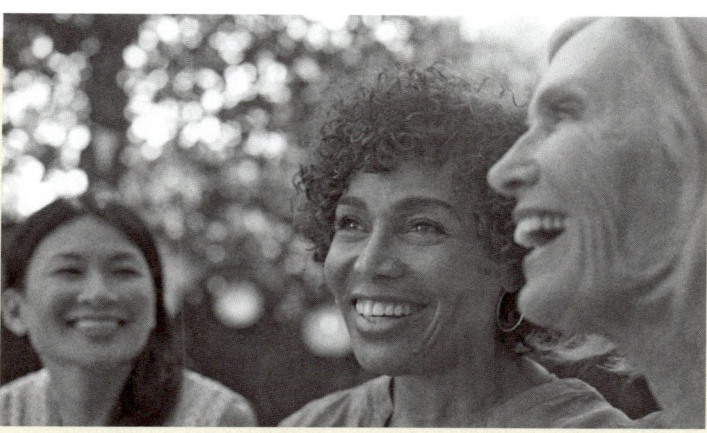

Researchers have long known that people who are lonely and socially isolated have more health problems, particularly as they age. They have a higher incidence of everything from colds and flu to heart disease, depression, Alzheimer's, and even aggressive cancers. A variety of explanations have been offered, including behavioral ones—for example, that people who lack a network of close friends or family have no one to help motivate them to eat right and exercise. But now it appears that there may be another reason. It seems that loneliness causes white blood cells to be more active, leading to higher levels of inflammation.

For a study published in *Proceedings of the National Academy of Sciences*, researchers at the University of California, Los Angeles, tracked 141 people for five years. They recorded "perceived loneliness" at regular intervals and also took blood samples to gauge both gene activity and levels of a key neurotransmitter involved in the fight-or-flight response. The results clearly showed that loneliness was correlated with increased activity of inflammatory genes. It also went hand in hand with the dampened antiviral response (specifically, lower levels of interferon) typically found in the fight-or-flight setting. In short, different parts of the immune system were reacting in different ways—both of them to the detriment of people experiencing loneliness—even after the researchers accounted for other potential contributors to inflammation.

---

handle on your sleep, and address your everyday stressors, the less time harmful substances will have to accumulate in your body and increase your risk for chronic diseases. Incorporating the strategies discussed in this chapter into your daily life will gradually become so routine that in time, you will engage in them without having to consciously think about what you eat or whether you are going to exercise—these activities will simply have become old, and very good, habits.

If you've been following a pro-inflammatory lifestyle for decades and are struggling to break the cycle, a visit to your primary care provider for a check-up can be helpful. Go over your diet, exercise, sleep, and other lifestyle habits to identify areas for improvement. Assess your family history for potential risks like heart disease or autoimmune disease that could be in your future. And make sure you've had all of the routine tests that could highlight a potential problem, including tests for high blood pressure, cholesterol, and blood sugar.

Remember that anti-inflammatory living is a process. It can take time for you to adjust to a new and healthier routine, especially if you're fond of eating fast food, spending a lot of time on the couch, or smoking. Work incrementally, making small changes that you can manage. If you are new to exercise, walk 10 minutes a day for the first couple of weeks, then increase the time to 20 minutes, and then 30 minutes. Swap out one order of French fries for a salad each week, then replace one soda with a glass of sparkling water. As you make improvements to your lifestyle, check back in with your doctor. Once you see how these adjustments have affected your health in the form of lowered blood pressure, better cholesterol levels, healthier weight, reduced markers of inflammation, and improvements in diseases like diabetes and arthritis, you will realize that the results were well worth the effort you put in.

Inflammation and your heart

The single biggest killer of Americans isn't cancer, diabetes, injuries, or lung disease. It is heart trouble. According to the CDC, one in every four deaths is directly attributable to heart disease, which adds up to nearly 650,000 lives lost each year. Given the enormous human toll, researchers and doctors feel a particularly strong imperative to find the underlying causes and contributing factors of heart disease, and address them.

The most common type of heart disease, coronary artery disease, stems from the buildup of fatty, cholesterol-laden plaque inside the arteries of the heart. Doctors used to view coronary artery disease as simply a "plumbing problem." They theorized that a lifetime of eating fatty foods left globs of cholesterol on the inner surface of the blood vessels. Eventually, this sediment blocked blood flow, leading to a heart attack. In recent years, a more nuanced understanding has emerged, in which chronic inflammation plays a pivotal role in each step of the disease process.

The underpinnings of this new theory actually first appeared centuries ago. Greek physician Aretaeus of Cappadocia noticed inflammation in the aorta (the main artery carrying blood away from the heart) in the first century. But in recent years, new imaging techniques, coupled with advances in molecular biology, expanded our understanding.

Scientists now realize that when particles of LDL (bad) cholesterol infiltrate the innermost layers of the artery walls, which are lined with endothelial cells, inflammatory cells of various types bind to these cells and begin the inflammatory process (see Figure 8, page 39). The immune system views the plaque as a foreign substance, and initiates a response to wall off the plaque from the blood flow. Cytokines send out the alert to phagocytes, which rush to the site to gobble up the offending plaque.

As the phagocytes consume cholesterol particles, layers of fat and cellular debris build up within the artery lining. This causes the artery wall to thicken and stiffen, narrowing the channel for blood flow. Plaques in the arteries are covered by a layer of tissue known as a fibrous cap. If this cap pops open, the plaque can rupture, spilling its contents into the bloodstream. Platelets and other blood cells attach to the injury and form a clot, which can eventually grow large enough to block the flow of blood. If the clot blocks blood flow in a vessel that feeds the heart, it can trigger a heart attack. Or it might break off and travel through the bloodstream, into smaller and smaller blood vessels, ultimately getting stuck in one. If it becomes embedded in a vessel to the brain, it can set off the most common type of stroke. Either is a potentially life-threatening development.

Testing for inflammation

Signs of inflammation serve as a warning of your heart risks (as can gum disease; see "Gum disease and cardiovascular disease," page 40). Looking for markers of inflammation in your blood is one way for your doctor to assess your risk. The only inflammatory marker that is commonly tested for to assess cardiovascular risk is C-reactive protein (CRP), a substance your liver produces in response to inflammation within your body. Doctors test for CRP with a high-sensitivity blood test (known as an hsCRP test). A level lower than 1 milligram per liter (mg/L) means you are at low risk; 1 to 3 mg/L indicates average risk; and 3 mg/L means you are at high risk for cardiovascular disease, heart attack, and stroke. Medicare and most other insurers will cover the cost of the test, provided that your doctor recommends it based on your personal and family history of heart disease or other risk factors. If your CRP level is high, your doctor may order more tests to look for the cause of inflammation, and you may need to institute heart-protective lifestyle changes or start taking medication to manage your risks.

Continued on page 40

Figure 8: From healthy artery to heart attack

Heart attacks are not just the result of a buildup of fatty plaque in the arteries. Inflammation, triggered by damage to the inner lining of an artery, sets off the steady growth of atherosclerotic plaque. If a plaque suddenly ruptures, it can lead to a heart attack.

STAGE 1: Excess LDL passes through the artery

Cholesterol travels in the bloodstream within spherical particles called lipoproteins. About two-thirds of blood cholesterol is in the form of low-density lipoprotein (LDL), often called "bad" cholesterol, because excess LDL leaves the blood and lodges in the artery walls. Having high LDL increases your risk for atherosclerosis.

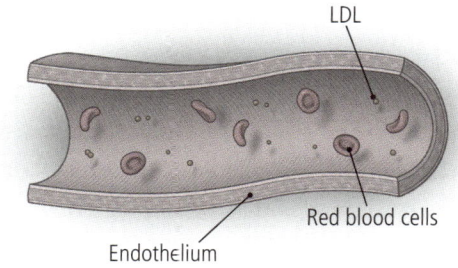

STAGE 2: Plaque builds up and the artery narrows

LDL cholesterol lodges in the artery wall, where it triggers a harmful sequence of events. The immune system recognizes the resulting plaque as a foreign substance and launches an attack on it. White blood cells travel to the site and engulf LDL cholesterol in the artery wall. These cells then enlarge and transform into fat-laden foam cells.

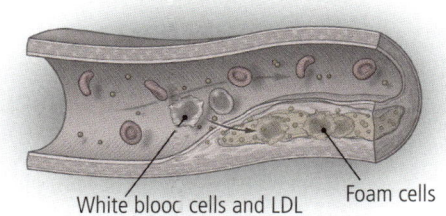

STAGE 3: A fibrous cap tops the plaque

As foam cells die, they release a soft, fatty substance that provokes further inflammation. Smooth muscle cells in the artery wall enlarge and multiply, forming a cap over the whole mess and adding to the bulk of the plaque. Some large plaques may be contained mainly within the vessel wall, while others can extend into the interior of the artery, limiting blood flow and delivery of oxyben. The bigger the plaque, the more blood flow is restricted.

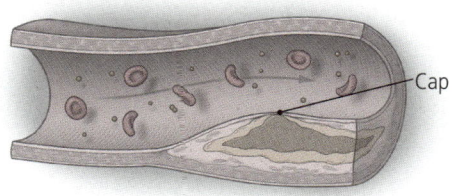

STAGE 4: The plaque ruptures

About three of every four heart attacks occur because of plaque rupture. But is it not necessarily the large plaques that are most dangerous. Large plaques are often covered by thick, fibrous caps that resist breaking apart. By contrast, smaller plaques may be active, dynamic lesions teeming with inflammatory cells and may have very thin caps that rupture easily.

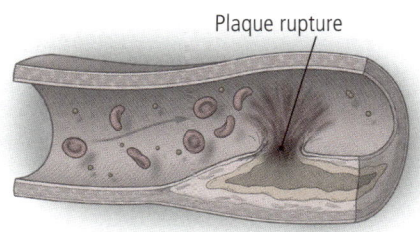

STAGE 5: A clot blocks the artery

Once a plaque ruptures, a protein called tissue factor is released into the bloodstream, where it attracts platelets. The platelets stick to the disrupted plaque, triggering proteins in the blood to start clotting. The result is a thrombus—a clot made up of red blood cells, platelets, and other material—that can be large enough to prevent blood from reaching the heart cells downstream. Deprived of blood and oxygen, a portion of the heart muscle dies.

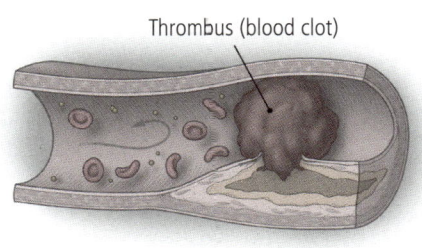

Continued from page 38

Controlling inflammation to shield the heart

Since the discovery that inflammation plays a role in heart disease, researchers have been on a quest to learn whether drugs that combat inflammatory processes might prevent heart attacks and other cardiovascular events.

In 2008, the JUPITER study found that, in older adults with elevated levels of inflammatory markers in their blood who did not have high cholesterol, treatment with a cholesterol-lowering statin drug lowered the risk for heart attacks and strokes. However, it was not clear from the study whether these effects were simply a byproduct of the statins' ability to lower cholesterol or due to other factors, such as reduced inflammation. Evidence suggests that statins may have anti-inflammatory and antioxidant properties that protect the artery walls against damage from cholesterol. They may also

- protect heart and blood vessel cells directly by speeding DNA repair and slowing cell death
- help arteries widen to carry more blood to the heart muscle and other tissues
- stabilize cholesterol-laden plaques, reducing the chance that they will rupture and trigger heart attacks
- inhibit platelets, thus helping to prevent artery-blocking blood clots
- reduce blood viscosity or "thickness," perhaps easing blood flow through partially blocked arteries.

A major turning point in doctors' thinking about treatment came in 2019, with the results of the CANTOS study. Researchers randomly assigned more than 10,000 people who had high CRP levels and who'd had a heart attack to take the monoclonal antibody drug canakinumab (Ilaris) in one of three doses, or a placebo (inactive treatment). Canakinumab targets the cytokine interleukin-1 beta to bring down inflammation. Participants who took the drug were 15% less likely to have another heart attack or stroke, showing that reducing inflammation, even without lowering cholesterol levels, can significantly affect heart disease risk. Canakinumab isn't widely prescribed for lowering inflammation, in part because of its high cost and side effects, which include a higher risk for infections. Studies are investigating whether other, potentially cheaper and safer anti-inflammatory drugs might similarly reduce heart risks. As noted, statins—the most widely prescribed cholesterol-lowering drugs—also have anti-inflammatory effects.

That said, doctors regard a healthy lifestyle as the first line of defense against heart disease (see the Special Section, "Combating chronic inflammation with lifestyle changes," page 29). Lifestyle measures like a plant-based diet, exercise, and smoking cessation remain the cornerstones of cardiovascular health, recommended by major organizations like the American Heart Association—and all of these strategies help combat inflammation. ♥

Gum disease and cardiovascular disease

Gum disease begins with the sticky plaque that builds up around your teeth. This is not the same as the fat- and cholesterol-laden plaque that lines your arteries when you have heart disease, but the two conditions are more closely related than you might think. People with gum disease face a 50% higher risk of a heart attack than people without gum disease.

Some of the association between the two conditions may reflect shared risk factors. For example, people who indulge in large quantities of sugary sodas and junk foods are more prone to both inflamed gums (gingivitis) and clogged arteries. Smoking is also linked to both gum disease and heart disease. Yet there is growing evidence that gum disease may be its own independent risk factor for cardiovascular problems. One theory is that the same bacteria that grow in the gums spread through the bloodstream and provoke inflammation in the arteries around the heart. As evidence, researchers have discovered bacteria from the mouth in blood vessels far away.

Another possibility is that bodywide inflammation is to blame for both conditions. Research suggests that other systemic, inflammatory conditions may also be associated with gum disease, including type 2 diabetes, osteoporosis, and rheumatoid arthritis.

To date, there is no evidence that regular brushing and flossing will spare you from a heart attack. But given the possible connection, it just makes good sense to pay attention to your oral hygiene by brushing and flossing every day, seeing your dentist for twice-yearly cleanings, and not smoking.

Inflammation and your brain

When you stub your toe or cut a finger, the resulting inflammation is rapid and obvious. Deep inside your brain, inflammation can be more gradual and much harder to detect. Yet the effects of long-term inflammation on the brain can be much more destructive than a visible toe or finger injury.

Researchers have linked brain inflammation to the development of neurodegenerative conditions like Alzheimer's and Parkinson's, as well as to mental health conditions ranging from depression to schizophrenia. Now they are trying to understand what mechanisms underlie the connection, and how combating inflammation might protect this vulnerable organ.

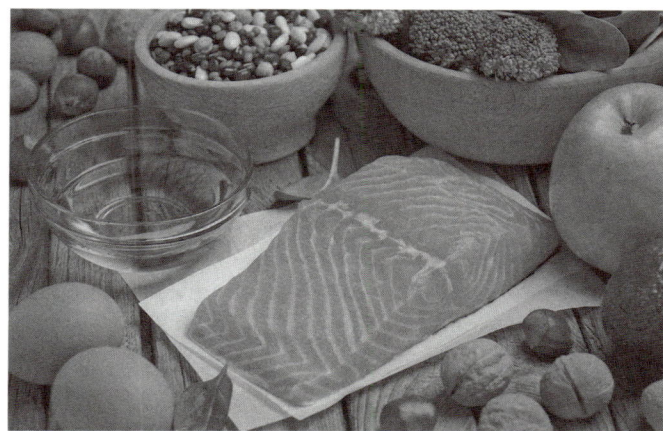

The MIND diet, developed to reduce the risk of dementia, emphasizes leafy greens, other vegetables, nuts, berries, and fish such as salmon. The diet is associated with a slower rate of cognitive decline.

The brain's defense system

For protective purposes, the brain has a different set of defenses than the rest of the body. Because an all-out assault by the immune system against bacteria or toxins could prove devastating to sensitive brain and nerve tissues, brain immunity takes a decidedly gentler approach. Yet when the injury is extreme, such as in the case of a stroke (see page 42) or sepsis (see "Infections and brain fog," below right), the inflammatory response may be more severe and more closely resemble the response elsewhere in the body.

The brain's immune system is termed the neuroimmune system. Its first line of defense is the blood-brain barrier, which separates the blood coursing through blood vessels of the brain from the surrounding cells and tissues. In other parts of the body, blood vessels are lined with endothelial cells, which are spaced to allow substances to move relatively easily in and out of the vessels. In the brain, the barrier is far less permeable. It allows in oxygen, glucose, and other nutrients the brain needs, but it bars entry to germs and toxins in the bloodstream that might damage brain cells.

The next line of defense is a specialized team of macrophages called microglia, which are often referred to as scavenger cells. They constantly scan the brain for signs of injury or infection. When they detect either one, microglia multiply, release inflammatory substances, and engulf germs, damaged cells, and other debris.

Microglia are the central players in the inflammatory response in the brain (neuroinflammation). As in the rest of the body, this process was intended to serve as a protective mechanism. But when the activation of microglia is significant (such as after a traumatic brain injury or stroke) or when it becomes chronic (as in the case of an illness like Alzheimer's disease or multiple sclerosis), the inflammatory substances that are released can have detrimental effects, and may ultimately lead to cognitive decline (dementia) and depression. Microglia have also been implicated in other neurodegenerative disorders, including Parkinson's disease, ischemic stroke, and traumatic brain injury.

Infections and brain fog

If you've ever come down with a nasty cold or bout of the flu, you may have experienced the temporary "brain fog" that often accompanies such infections.

Experts have surmised that neuroinflammation during an infection contributes to this swift and dramatic drop in cognition.

There are several theories about how inflammation might lead to these mental effects. One study found that inflammation related to an infection specifically affects areas of the brain that normally keep you alert, which could explain the brain fog some people experience when ill.

Despite the blood-brain barrier, the brain is vulnerable to inflammation elsewhere in the body. A dramatic example of this is the rapid mental decline that occurs in people with sepsis, a life-threatening condition in which an overwhelming infection causes multiple organ dysfunction. In sepsis, an overly robust immune response (known as a cytokine storm) creates widespread inflammation that leads to such symptoms as severe weakness, trouble breathing, and abnormal function of the heart and other organs. Without swift treatment, the person dies. More than 80% of people with this extreme, whole-body response to infection develop delirium. Bodywide inflammation can disrupt communication between nerve cells and cause permanent damage to the brain's structure. Indeed, imaging studies have revealed damage to various parts of the brain in people with sepsis.

Even low-grade inflammation, if ongoing, might contribute to mental decline. A study published in 2019 in the journal *Neurology* assigned more than 12,000 middle-aged adults a composite score based on levels of four inflammatory markers in their blood. The participants' thinking and memory skills were tested at the beginning of the study, six to nine years later, and at the end of the 20-year study. People who started with the highest inflammation scores had nearly 8% more cognitive decline compared with those who began with the lowest scores. The authors say it is possible that chronic inflammation is not a cause of mental decline, but rather a marker of or a response to brain diseases that cause such decline. But they add that inflammation may still be a possible target for treatments.

Stroke

A stroke can be both a result of inflammation and a cause of it. The same inflammatory processes that damage arteries and contribute to heart attacks can also harm the blood vessels that supply brain cells with oxygen- and nutrient-rich blood. Up to 85% of strokes are the type called ischemic stroke, which occurs when a blood clot or clump of plaque material blocks a blood vessel in the brain. (The other type, hemorrhagic stroke, occurs when a blood vessel in the brain bursts, causing bleeding into the brain.)

Starved of blood and nutrients, neurons (brain cells) begin to die rapidly, at an estimated rate of 1.9 million cells per minute. As these brain cells die, they release molecules called DAMPs (see "Act 2: Innate immunity," page 8)—signals that activate and recruit inflammatory cells like neutrophils, T cells, macrophages, and phagocytes to the area. These cells release their own signals to call in even more inflammatory reinforcements to the response.

During the initial phase of the stroke, which may last anywhere from a few minutes to several hours, the production of cytokines and reactive oxygen species ramps up. Inflammatory mediators widen the blood vessels and increase permeability of the blood-brain barrier. Additional blood, as well as more of the immune system's defense cells, rush to the site of the injury.

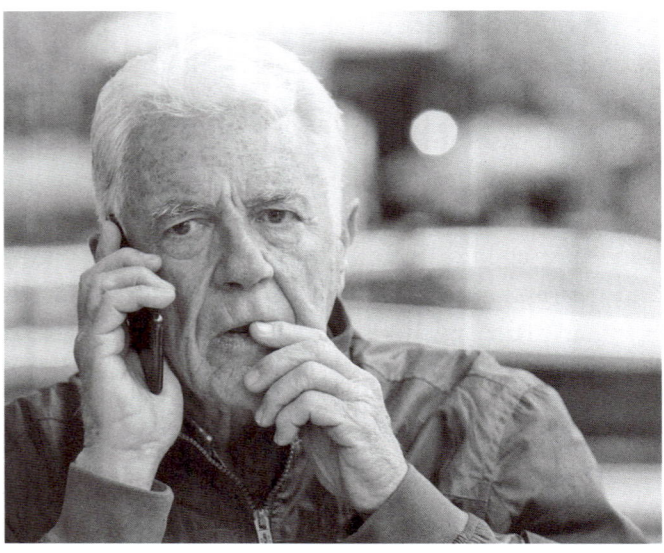

Brain fog may be the result of inflammation elsewhere in the body. One study found that inflammation related to an infection affects specific areas of the brain that normally keep you alert.

Microglia also appear. They clean up the stroke damage by engulfing cellular debris. Yet their actions aren't all positive. Microglia also release pro-inflammatory cytokines like TNF and interleukin-1 that may hasten the death of even more neurons.

Stroke-related inflammation has multiple deleterious effects on the brain.

For one, it may contribute to post-stroke depression (PSD), which afflicts about one-third of stroke survivors (see "Depression," page 44). PSD typically begins within a few months after a stroke, and it can last for two to three years afterward. Because depression may make recovery from a stroke more difficult, people with PSD are at increased risk for a worse prognosis or death.

In addition, neuroinflammation may contribute to post-stroke cognitive impairment or even dementia. Up to one-third of stroke survivors will go on to develop dementia—most often vascular dementia, but sometimes Alzheimer's disease or both together. In part, that's because stroke and dementia share risk factors like advancing age, high blood pressure, obesity, and smoking. But the brain changes induced by a stroke may also directly contribute to the brain atrophy and buildup of abnormal beta-amyloid proteins in Alzheimer's (see "Dementia, including Alzheimer's disease," above right).

Major research efforts are focused on understanding the underlying mechanisms of post-stroke cognitive impairment and dementia. Most recently, the National Institutes of Health awarded $39 million to a new national network of academic centers, led by Harvard, that will examine various factors, including neuroinflammation.

Standard treatment for an ischemic stroke today is medicine or surgery to break up or remove the clot and restore blood flow—preferably within a few hours of when the stroke occurs. Doctors then use anti-clotting drugs and other medications to control risk factors and prevent a recurrence. Researchers are investigating whether anti-inflammatory drugs may improve outcomes by helping reduce inflammation after a stroke. So far, this treatment has shown promise in animal studies, but its effects have not yet been confirmed in humans.

Dementia, including Alzheimer's disease

Many Americans fear Alzheimer's disease—the most common form of dementia—more than strokes, heart attacks, and even cancer. The potential loss of your own history, your memory of loved ones, and your ability to care for yourself makes Alzheimer's a formidable and fearsome adversary. The statistics only add to the sense of anxiety: nearly six million Americans currently live with Alzheimer's, and by the year 2050, that number is expected to surge to nearly 14 million. The rising number of dementia patients underscores the need to better understand the mechanisms that underlie this disease and to address them with new treatments.

The hallmarks of Alzheimer's disease are the sticky amyloid plaques and twisted tangles of tau protein that are found in the brains of people with the disease. What scientists don't yet understand is what mechanisms are behind the deposits of these abnormal proteins and whether they actually contribute to dementia. One area of increasing interest is inflammation.

One of the first pathological changes in Alzheimer's disease is the accumulation of beta-amyloid in brain tissue. As the disease takes hold, brain cells begin to die, and levels of neurotransmitters, which carry messages between billions of neurons, decline. Many of the connections between brain neurons, so crucial for memory and other mental functions, also disappear.

The formation of beta-amyloid plaques appears to initiate an immune response within the brain tissue. Microglia cells amass around the plaques in an attempt to eradicate the unwanted protein and clear away damaged cells. But unlike a virus or bacterium, plaques are not easily vanquished. They persist and continue to taunt the immune system into constant and unrelenting action. As the battle rages on, cytokines and other inflammatory chemicals continue to be released, inflicting collateral damage on healthy brain cells. Inflammation also boosts the activity of a substance called beta-amyloid cleaving enzyme, which in a vicious cycle ramps up beta-amyloid production.

Inflammation also leads to the accumulation of another abnormal protein called tau. Tau is a structural component of cells that helps stabilize the microscopic tubes (called microtubules) that allow for the transport of molecules from one end of the cell to another. In Alzheimer's disease, however, tau collapses into threads that eventually form tangles. These tangles further interfere with the neurons' ability to communicate. If scientists can firmly establish the role inflammation plays in the development of Alzheimer's disease, the hope is that they will be able to find treatments to stop the progression of, or even prevent, cognitive decline and dementia.

Inflammation is also deeply involved in the second leading form of dementia, vascular dementia. This type results from damage to blood vessels in the brain, which typically involves an inflammatory process. Strokes (see page 42) are one cause of vascular dementia. Vascular dementia can also stem from multiple small strokes or, most commonly, from chronic damage to many tiny blood vessels in the brain. In addition, inflammation can worsen the damage from strokes.

Inflammation also appears to contribute to the increased risk for dementia among people who suffer a traumatic brain injury (TBI). TBI is one of the leading risk factors for dementia later in life; a severe head injury can increase the risk for Alzheimer's fourfold. It also contributes to the risk for Parkinson's disease, multiple sclerosis, and amyotrophic lateral sclerosis (ALS).

After a TBI, the brain launches a series of events termed the secondary injury cascade, which includes neuroinflammation, the loss of neurons, and the production and deposit of beta-amyloid. The activation of microglia also contributes to the generation of beta-amyloid plaques. Beta-amyloid and tau both increase in the brain of someone who's had a TBI, sometimes within hours after the injury. The buildup of these proteins plays a role in the death of neurons after the injury, although the exact mechanisms linking TBI and dementia are still unclear.

Depression

Like all medical knowledge, the understanding of depression has undergone a seismic shift over the centuries. In the earliest accounts, unearthed from ancient Mesopotamia, depression and other mental illnesses were seen as the result of demonic possession. The demons needed to be exorcised for those afflicted to find relief. Today, scientists have come to the realization that depression has biological roots.

One interesting development has been the discovery that depression shares many of the same characteristics, risk factors, and symptoms as immune-based inflammatory responses. We know that low mood, appetite loss, sleep disturbances, trouble concentrating, and a lack of energy are clear hallmarks of depression, but these are also signs of inflammation. Many of the same risk factors that make people more vulnerable to depression—like stress, obesity, and eating a highly processed diet—also put them at risk for heart disease and other inflammatory conditions.

Chronic inflammatory diseases like rheumatoid arthritis, inflammatory bowel disease, atherosclerotic heart disease, and diabetes have all been linked to an increased risk for depression. Doctors once believed that depression was the natural result of living with one of these chronic and painful diseases, but they now recognize that the relationship is more complex than that. The inflammation these diseases share is central to the connection between them.

People who've been diagnosed with depression have higher levels of pro-inflammatory cytokines and other markers of inflammation in their blood. Studies suggest that when someone without any signs of depression has elevated inflammatory markers, he or she may be at higher risk of developing depression in the future.

Further evidence of the connection between inflammation and depression comes from research on cytokines. In studies, animals that were given cytokines became lethargic, withdrawn, and uninterested in food or sex—familiar symptoms to anyone who has grappled with depression.

A similar effect has been seen in people with hepatitis C who are treated with interferon drugs—manufactured versions of the natural cytokines known as interferons. This type of drug was once a staple of treatment for hepatitis C because it "interferes" with the virus's ability to replicate; however, it is far less effective and causes more side effects than newer treatments.

When people with hepatitis receive interferon, they commonly become tired and achy, as if they had come down with the flu. (In fact, when people are infected with the influenza virus, it is cytokines that produce the overwhelming feeling of fatigue that keeps them confined to their bed for days.) Continued treatment with interferon often leads to an increase in depression and anxiety symptoms. Depression triggered by interferon administration is typically treated with antidepressants, just like other types of depression; however, when it's severe, interferon may have to be stopped.

In recent years, findings by investigators doing laboratory research on cells suggest that inflammation may increase depression risk by suppressing the birth of new brain cells (called neurogenesis) and hastening the death of existing brain cells (called apoptosis). This decrease in neurogenesis is believed to be an important factor contributing to the development of depression.

Now the hunt is on to see if anti-inflammatory therapies may have a role in treating depression. Given that about one-third of people with depression don't respond to traditional antidepressant drugs, there is a pressing need to find alternatives. NSAIDs and the antibiotic tetracycline are among the candidates under investigation. So far, it has not been clear whether these drugs have any real effect on depressive symptoms. One potential downside to them is that they may actually block the beneficial effects of antidepressant medications. And because NSAIDs come with risks like increased bleeding and heart problems, they are currently not recommended for treating or preventing depression.

Fighting inflammation to protect the brain

There is a big effort under way in the pharmaceutical industry to find drugs that calm inflammation in the brain to treat a variety of diseases, including Alzheimer's. Some studies have suggested that people who take NSAIDs like aspirin or ibuprofen have a lower risk of developing Alzheimer's. But so far, the results of research on anti-inflammatory therapies for combating dementia have been disappointing.

One of the most promising of those therapies was the antibiotic minocycline (Minocin). In addition to its ability to fight a variety of infectious agents, this drug has anti-inflammatory and neuroprotective properties, as well as the ability to slip relatively easily across the blood-brain barrier. Research had suggested that minocycline, along with transcranial magnetic stimulation (which uses magnetic fields to stimulate neurons in the brain), might help neurons recover and regenerate after a stroke. Yet in a two-year study, minocycline treatment at two different doses (200 and 400 mg) did not slow cognitive decline in people with mild Alzheimer's disease, and it caused side effects.

A two-year investigation of an NSAID among people at high risk for Alzheimer's disease had similarly disappointing results. Twice-daily treatment with naproxen did not slow cognitive decline, and it caused significant side effects like gastrointestinal and cardiovascular problems.

Other investigators are combining the NSAID ibuprofen with cromolyn, a drug normally used (under the brand name Intal) to target inflammation in the lungs to treat asthma. In studies of mice, cromolyn treatment has been shown to reduce deposits of beta-amyloid plaques. It remains to be seen whether the drug might help stave off dementia in humans.

A brain-healthy diet could also help. Most beneficial to the brain may be the MIND Diet, which is a cross between the Mediterranean diet (see page 31) and the low-sodium, high-produce DASH diet, with emphasis on certain brain-healthy foods such as berries and leafy greens. The diet was developed by Martha Clare Morris, a nutritional epidemiologist at Rush University Medical Center. A 2016 study found that the diet helped reduce the risk of developing Alzheimer's during a 4.5-year period. And a 2018 study found that it was associated with a substantially slower rate of cognitive decline in stroke survivors.

Timing might be everything when it comes to stemming the inflammation that leads to cognitive decline. Anti-inflammatory strategies may be most effective when it is started before dementia develops, to help prevent the condition. ▼

Inflammation and metabolic disease

We are in the midst of an obesity epidemic. Worldwide, more than 1.9 billion people are considered overweight, and more than 650 million are obese. The prevalence of obesity has doubled since 1980. And with it, complications like type 2 diabetes and metabolic syndrome (which sets the stage for heart disease) have become exceedingly common and have taken a devastating toll on the world's population.

Both are metabolic problems, meaning they involve the dysregulation of metabolism (the cellular processes of converting protein, carbohydrates, and fats into energy and converting stored energy into growth). Because these processes occur throughout the body, metabolic problems can affect multiple organs—the pancreas, liver, heart, muscles, and brain among them.

Over the past two decades, researchers have begun to draw a clear line connecting excess weight with metabolic dysregulation and inflammation—specifically, a special kind of constant, low-grade inflammation that scientists have named metabolically triggered inflammation, or meta-inflammation. It plays a role in both type 2 diabetes and metabolic syndrome.

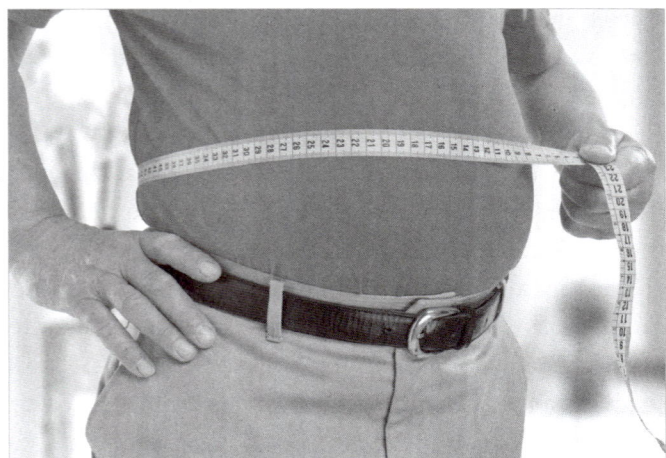

Excess weight, especially around the belly, is linked to inflammation. The fat cells there are particularly active metabolically, churning out a variety of pro-inflammatory compounds.

Type 2 diabetes

Doctors have long observed that obesity and diabetes tend to go hand in hand. So strong is the correlation that some experts refer to the combination of the two as "diabesity." Both involve inflammation. Recently, the role of chronic inflammation in the disease process has begun to come into focus. Inflammation is an important trigger that sets type 2 diabetes into motion once other preconditions are in place—for example, excess weight, a poor diet, and a sedentary lifestyle. Inflammation also is a major contributor to many of the disease's complications, including heart attacks, strokes, and kidney disease.

What is diabetes?

Diabetes is a disease marked by high blood sugar. Normally when you eat, as your body breaks down carbohydrates from food into sugar (glucose), your blood sugar level rises. In response, the pancreas releases the hormone insulin, which enables muscle, fat, and liver cells to take up sugar from the bloodstream to either use for energy or store for future use. Diabetes disrupts this normal cycle.

Two different forms of the disease exist. Type 1 diabetes (see page 27) is an autoimmune disease. The immune system attacks and destroys insulin-producing cells in the pancreas, and the resulting lack of insulin eventually leads to high blood sugar.

Type 2 diabetes, which account for 95% of diabetes cases, also results in high blood sugar, but the underlying disease process is different. In type 2 diabetes, the body still makes insulin, but cells throughout the body don't respond appropriately to it—a problem known as insulin resistance. The pancreas produces more insulin in an attempt to overcome this resistance. After a few years of struggling to keep up with the body's ever-increasing insulin demand, the pancreatic cells become increasingly exhausted. At that point, in addition to insulin resistance, there is also too little insulin. This combination leads to the consistently elevated blood sugar that's characteristic of diabetes.

Because diabetes affects levels of glucose in the bloodstream, complications may develop throughout the body if blood sugar isn't kept well under control. Diabetes can damage the eyes and increase the risk for retinal disease (retinopathy), cataracts, and glaucoma. It can damage the kidneys, which filter the blood, and lead to kidney disease. It can damage nerves (a condition called neuropathy), causing pain, numbness, and tingling. And it can damage blood vessels that feed the heart and brain, increasing the risk for heart disease and strokes. People with type 2 diabetes develop cardiovascular disease earlier (perhaps a decade earlier) and more severely than do people without diabetes.

The role of fat and inflammation

People tend to think of fat cells as inert storage depots for calories. On the contrary, fat cells are metabolically active. Fat produces a variety of pro-inflammatory substances, like TNF and interleukins. A number of these substances interfere with the functioning of insulin, including TNF and a compound called resistin, so named because it contributes to insulin resistance.

Because the fat that accumulates around your middle is the most metabolically active, having an "apple" shape (in which you carry extra fat around your waist) is more dangerous than having a "pear" shape (in which excess fat settles around your hips).

Not all the products of fat cells are harmful, however. Fat cells also make a compound called adiponectin, which *reduces* insulin resistance. Unfortunately, the more excess weight you have—particularly, the more visceral (belly) fat—the more resistin and the less adiponectin you produce.

That's not the only problem with excess weight. When you put on pounds, fat can accumulate in the liver, muscles, and other organs. In the liver, the storage of excess fat (hepatic steatosis, or fatty liver) can lead to inflammation and cause non-alcoholic fatty liver disease (NAFLD). NAFLD is becoming the most common cause of cirrhosis and liver failure requiring transplantation.

A similar process is at play elsewhere in the body, contributing to some of the complications of type 2 diabetes. For example, in the arteries, the release of pro-inflammatory substances helps set the stage for cardiovascular disease, which is linked to obesity and type 2 diabetes.

Diabetes is also associated with a higher risk of several cancers, including those of the liver, pancreas, ovary, colon, lung, bladder, and breast. There are a few possible explanations for this link. First, cancer and diabetes share important risk factors, such as aging, obesity, a sedentary lifestyle, and a diet high in fat and refined carbohydrates. Second, biochemical changes associated with diabetes—such as insulin resistance, high blood sugar, and inflammation—may also contribute to the development of cancer. This evidence is still preliminary, so more research is needed.

Metabolic syndrome

Metabolic syndrome is a combination of conditions that increase the risk of heart disease, type 2 diabetes, stroke, and cancer. These conditions include abdominal obesity, high blood pressure (hypertension), abnormal cholesterol and triglyceride levels, and impaired glucose tolerance (difficulty controlling blood sugar levels). In recent years, researchers have discovered that inflammation contributes to its complications.

Metabolic syndrome, obesity, and type 2 diabetes are interconnected. All three of these conditions are linked by genetics, overeating, an unhealthy diet, and lack of exercise. And all of them are marked by a chronic state of inflammation in the body.

Scientists do not completely understand all of the factors involved in metabolic syndrome, but they do have a few theories. One area of focus is on mitochondria—the energy-producing organelles in each of our cells. Mitochondria do more than just generate energy. They also play an important role in many cellular functions, including helping cells multiply when they are needed, and die off when they are not needed. Mitochondrial dysfunction has been linked to insulin resistance, and it can damage both cells and the organs in which they reside.

Chronic low-grade inflammation has been identified as both a cause and a consequence of metabolic syndrome. People with metabolic syndrome have higher-than-normal levels of inflammatory markers like CRP (see "Testing for inflammation," page 38) and TNF, particularly in the liver, intestines, and adipose tissue. These markers are also predictors of insulin resistance, type 2 diabetes, and cardiovascular disease.

Combating inflammation in metabolic diseases

Today, the first-line treatments for metabolic syndrome and type 2 diabetes are lifestyle interventions directed at weight loss. In particular, doctors recommend a diet rich in fruits and vegetables, whole grains, and low-fat diary, and low in saturated fat and sugar (see "Eat to beat inflammation," page 29). Increased activity is also recommended—in part, because movement demands energy, which in turn makes cells absorb glucose more efficiently. To some extent, exercise also helps with weight loss, though it is more effective for maintaining weight loss than achieving it in the first place. These strategies are naturally anti-inflammatory, and together they have been shown to prevent the development and progression of both metabolic syndrome and type 2 diabetes.

When it comes to medication, the current approach is to treat each component of these conditions—high blood sugar, high blood pressure, abnormal cholesterol, and so forth—separately, with a different targeted drug. Yet researchers are discovering that some of the drugs doctors are already using to manage these diseases also serve double duty by dampening inflammation.

For example, many of the medications doctors currently prescribe to control soaring blood sugar in people with type 2 diabetes simultaneously reduce levels of inflammation. Medications with anti-inflammatory effects include insulin; metformin (Glucophage); and GLP-1 receptor agonists like exenatide (Byetta) and liraglutide (Victoza). Some have even been shown to reduce inflammatory markers in the blood. Metformin also has been shown to alter the composition of the microbiome (see "The role of the microbiome in inflammatory diseases," page 24), which may play a role in the development of metabolic syndrome and related diseases.

More recently, researchers have been investigating whether standard anti-inflammatory drugs might have some value in treating diabetes. Although the early studies of anti-inflammatory agents for diabetes treatment have generally been negative, they remain under active investigation.

Some of the same drugs used to harness inflammation in autoimmune diseases like rheumatoid arthritis—including methotrexate and biologic medications (see "Taming inflammation to treat autoimmune diseases," page 28)—may also have potential for *preventing* diabetes. For example, people with inflammatory diseases who were given TNF inhibitors showed better blood sugar control and a lower incidence of type 2 diabetes. More research is needed in this area.

Drugs aren't the only way to control inflammation in diabetes and metabolic syndrome. In addition to lifestyle interventions, bariatric surgery is highly effective in promoting weight loss and thus reducing inflammation. In sleeve gastrectomy, the most common form of this procedure, part of the stomach is removed, limiting the amount of food the stomach can hold. Weight-loss surgery is recommended for people with type 2 diabetes who are severely obese (who have a body mass index of 40 or higher). Not only does this procedure result in significant weight loss, but within the following two years, up to 70% of people have improved metabolic measurements and have gone into remission from type 2 diabetes. Bariatric surgery also reduces levels of inflammatory markers in the blood and may lower the risk of heart attacks and strokes.

Inflammation and cancer

The largest single-year reduction in cancer deaths ever reported occurred in 2016–2017, thanks to advances in treatments and a reduction in smoking rates, according to the American Cancer Society. Yet cancer is an enemy not easily conquered. The rates of certain cancer diagnoses in the United States are still rising, particularly for melanoma, kidney, liver, and breast cancers. That is why searching for new methods to prevent and combat this disease remains of utmost importance.

When it comes to cancer development, the immune system is a double-edged sword. To begin with, it hunts down and destroys any abnormal cells in the body, including cancer cells. Without this action, we would succumb to far more cancers than we do. As cancer cells first begin to form small tumors, T cells of the immune system recognize and destroy them before they can grow too large and cause damage. This is called the "expansion" stage of the cancer-killing process. As cancer cells and immune cells battle, the cancer doesn't grow and essentially stays inactive. This is the "equilibrium" stage.

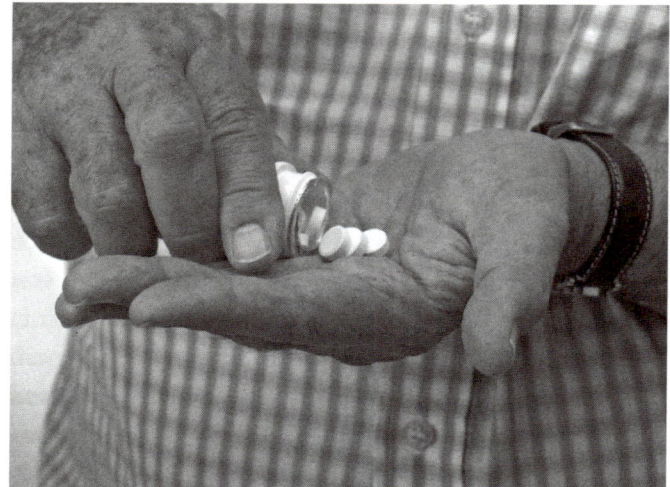

Good evidence suggests that aspirin and other nonsteroidal anti-inflammatory drugs have powerful anti-cancer properties. They block enzymes that play a role in pain and inflammation.

Cancer cells are wily adversaries, however. In time, they can develop genetic mutations, or changes, that enable them to become essentially invisible to the immune system and elude detection by T cells. These mutated cancer cells lose the molecules on their cell surface that help T cells recognize them. Cancer cells also learn how to disable immune cells and alter the environment in ways that make it too hostile for T cells to operate. This is called the "escape" stage, and it is the point at which cancer cells can again multiply, form tumors, and spread to other parts of the body.

When the immune system becomes the enemy

While your immune system unquestionably protects you against cancer, innate immunity (see "Act 2: Innate immunity," page 8) and inflammation also play central roles in driving tumor development. When infections, autoimmune responses, or conditions such as obesity go awry and cause chronic inflammation, that inflammation can over time promote the growth and replication of cancer cells.

Back in 1863, German physician Rudolf Virchow discovered leukocytes—white blood cells—in cancerous tissue. He was the first person to make a clear connection between inflammation and cancer, coming to the conclusion that cancer occurred as a result of inflammation that remained unchecked. But only recently have investigators identified chronic inflammation as a risk factor for cancer. In 1986, Harvard University pathologist and vascular researcher Harold Dvorak noticed some similarities between inflammation and cancer, including the proliferation of cells such as lymphocytes and macrophages, which are also activated at the site of injuries. At the time, he referred to tumors as "wounds that do not heal."

One of the clearest links between inflammation and cancer is evident in cancer-causing infections. In developing countries, nearly a quarter of cancers are caused by infections with pathogens like hepatitis B and C (liver cancer), human papillomavirus (cervical and anal cancers), and *H. pylori* bacteria (stomach cancer). Some viruses and bacteria directly cause cells to turn cancerous, while others produce a state of chronic inflammation, releasing pro-inflammatory substances that help cancers grow and thrive. HIV (the AIDS virus), which weakens the body's immune response to the point where it cannot defend against other infections, increases the risk of many types of cancer, including Kaposi's sarcoma, non-Hodgkin's lymphoma, and cervical cancer.

Inflammatory diseases also create an environment hospitable to cancer growth. People with inflammatory bowel disease (Crohn's disease or ulcerative colitis) are at increased risk for colon cancer, presumably because inflammation damages cells in their digestive tract to the point where they can turn cancerous. People with rheumatoid arthritis face about double the risk of developing non-Hodgkin's lymphoma. It is the disease itself that contributes to this increased risk. The same immune cells that become active and produce inflammation in rheumatoid arthritis—B cells and T cells—are the ones that turn malignant in lymphoma. People whose disease is poorly controlled—those with the greatest amount of inflammation—are at the highest risk for developing lymphoma.

Chronic inflammation increases cancer risk via several different mechanisms. For one thing, it damages DNA, causing mutations that allow cancer cells to multiply unchecked. Severe DNA damage activates an enzyme that not only repairs DNA, but also turns on the release of pro-inflammatory substances.

A state of chronic inflammation also creates a welcoming and nurturing environment in which cancer cells can replicate and spread further. The inflammatory process produces substances such as chemokines and other cytokines, growth factors, and free radicals that stimulate the proliferation of cancer cells while inhibiting their death. It also stimulates angiogenesis—the growth of new blood vessels that feed tumors. All of these processes help fuel cancer growth. Meanwhile, cancer cells themselves release substances that help to dampen the immune system's natural response against them.

Studies suggest that as many as 20% of cancers begin as a direct result of inflammation. And, many of the biggest cancer risk factors—including tobacco smoking, obesity, and alcohol use—are related to their ability to promote inflammation.

Targeting inflammation to fight cancer

Scientists have already begun to harness the protective effects of the immune system to help them fight cancer. Immunotherapy is a relatively new and exciting treatment that capitalizes on the immune system's ability to attack cancer. Immunotherapy uses substances engineered in a lab or made by the body to increase the immune system's capability to seek out and kill cancer.

Examples of immunotherapy drugs include monoclonal antibodies. Grown in the lab from clones of a single parent cell, these antibodies bind to receptors on the surface of cancer cells. Once they're bound to cancer cells, they alert the immune system to spring into action and destroy the cancer. Another group of immunotherapy drugs, called checkpoint inhibitors, block proteins called checkpoints, which normally keep an immune response from becoming too strong and which sometimes prevent T cells from killing cancer cells. These drugs take the brakes off the immune system response, cutting off pathways that cancer cells use to cloak themselves and evade attack. A third approach, known as chimeric antigen receptor (CAR) T-cell therapy, harvests T cells from the patient's own blood and genetically engineers them in a lab to add synthetic CAR receptors on their surface. These receptors allow the T cells to recognize a particular antigen on a cancer cell, making them more effective cancer-killing machines.

The hunt is on for cancer therapies that address the problem of inflammation. Several potential therapies targeting cytokines and immune cells are already under investigation in the laboratory. In studies using cell and mouse models of cancer, these inflammation-fighting therapies have significantly reduced the growth and spread of cancer.

But low-tech approaches that are already available may be useful, too, at least for helping to prevent cancer, and possibly for suppressing it in its early stages. Good evidence supports the idea that NSAIDs, especially aspirin, have powerful anti-cancer properties. These drugs work by blocking COX-1 and COX-2 enzymes, which are necessary for the production of prostaglandins, a group of hormones that play a role in triggering pain, inflammation, and fever during an infection or injury. Researchers have discovered that COX-2 enzymes are produced by colorectal cancer cells, as well as by almost every other type of cancer cell during the early stages when tumors form.

In a 2016 study published in *JAMA Neurology*, regular use of low-dose aspirin for a period of six years was associated with a significantly lower risk for cancer, especially cancers of the gastrointestinal tract. In other studies, NSAIDs not only reduced the risk of colorectal cancer, but they also reduced the number of existing polyps—precancerous growths in the colon—in people with the inherited disorder familial adenomatous polyposis (FAP), who are at significantly higher risk for colorectal cancer. Celecoxib is currently FDA-approved for preventing gastrointestinal cancers in people with FAP. The U.S. Preventive Services Task Force recommends that adults ages 50 to 59 who are at higher risk for cardiovascular disease take daily low-dose aspirin to prevent colorectal cancer as well as cardiovascular trouble. (For those ages 60 to 69, the decision should be individualized based on the person's heart disease and bleeding risks.)

Daily aspirin has the potential to prevent not only colorectal cancer, but also cancers of the esophagus, stomach, pancreas, lung, brain, and prostate. Long-term aspirin use may reduce cancer diagnoses and deaths by as much as 25%. The quandary patients and their doctors face when considering whether to prescribe daily NSAIDs is how to balance the cardiovascular and bleeding risks of these drugs with their ability to prevent cancer.

Other drugs are also being investigated for their preventive potential. Cholesterol-lowering statin drugs, which reduce levels of CRP and cytokines, appear to prevent the development of several cancers, including colorectal and breast cancers. The diabetes drug metformin (Glucophage) has been linked to a reduced risk for colon, breast, lung, prostate, and other cancers. Despite their potential, these drugs are not recommended at this time to prevent cancer. That approach is still experimental, and needs more validation in clinical trials to prove these drugs actually work against cancer.

One significant hurdle to overcome is the detrimental effect that tamping down inflammation might have on the immune response over all. As noted earlier, inflammation is not always a bad thing. You need the inflammatory response to protect you against infectious agents like bacteria and viruses, and to repair tissue damage. If you dampen it too much, those actions might be compromised. Harnessing the potential tumor-suppressing benefits of NSAIDs, statins, or metformin will require a deeper understanding of all the inflammatory mechanisms involved, so that therapies can target precisely the right ones.

A safer approach to cancer prevention focuses on lifestyle interventions like diet and exercise to tame inflammation. An estimated one in five cancer cases stems from a combination of excess weight, inactivity, poor nutrition, and excess alcohol use, all of which can contribute to inflammation, and all of which are preventable. In people who are obese, weight loss from bariatric surgery or other methods has been shown to reduce cancer risk. The use of omega-3 fatty acid supplements may also offer cancer protection to people who are obese, by bringing down inflammation in fat tissue. Reducing alcohol use and quitting smoking can similarly slow or prevent the development of cancer. As evidence, the recent reduction in cancer deaths coincided with lower smoking rates in the United States. All of these strategies are discussed in the Special Section beginning on page 29.

Whether you're aiming to prevent cancer or your focus is on heart disease, diabetes, or dementia, there are many reasons to adopt lifestyle measures that reduce low-grade chronic inflammation. With the understanding you've gained through this Special Health Report, we hope you can begin today to take measures to fight ongoing sources of inflammation—and live a longer, healthier life.

Resources

Organizations

Alzheimer's Association
800-272-3900 (toll-free)
www.alz.org

The Alzheimer's Association is the country's leading organization devoted to the care of people with this form of dementia. Its website offers a variety of resources and publications for both patients and caregivers, as well as information about its phone helpline and local support groups.

American Academy of Allergy, Asthma & Immunology (AAAAI)
414-272-6071
www.aaaai.org

This organization is made up of more than 7,000 allergists, immunologists, and other health specialists whose focus is on the treatment of allergies and immunologic diseases. AAAAI's website offers an overview of these conditions, as well as a comprehensive guide to the medicines used to treat them. It also offers a database of providers throughout the United States, searchable by city.

American Cancer Society
800-227-2345 (toll-free)
www.cancer.org

The American Cancer Society's website includes comprehensive information on each type of cancer, including causes, statistics, diagnosis, and treatment. It also offers tips on prevention and screening, as well as advice on paying for treatment.

American College of Rheumatology (ACR)
404-633-3777
www.rheumatology.org

This website for rheumatology professionals includes a consumer-friendly section, complete with overviews of rheumatic diseases such as arthritis. It includes information on what to do when you're newly diagnosed, how to manage your medications, and how to live better with these conditions.

American Diabetes Association (ADA)
800-DIABETES (800-342-2383, toll-free)
www.diabetes.org

This organization's mission is to improve the lives of people affected by diabetes. In addition to its advocacy work, the ADA offers a variety of tools and educational materials to help people with either type 1 or type 2 diabetes get a better handle on their disease. For anyone who hasn't yet been diagnosed, the ADA offers an online risk test that takes just 60 seconds.

Arthritis Foundation
404-872-7100
844-571-HELP (toll-free)
www.arthritis.org

This national nonprofit organization has local chapters in many states. The website has educational materials on arthritis, joint surgery, pain control, and standard and complementary therapies, as well as exercise videos and a directory of local offices and events. Local chapters may offer joint-health exercise classes.

National Heart, Lung, and Blood Institute (NHLBI)
877-NHLBI4U (877-645-2448, toll-free)
www.nhlbi.nih.gov

The NHLBI is the branch of the National Institutes of Health that deals with diseases related to the heart, lungs, and circulatory system. Its website contains information on heart disease, high blood pressure, and other conditions related to the heart and blood vessels.

National Institute of Arthritis and Musculoskeletal and Skin Diseases (NIAMS)
301-495-4484
877-226-4267 (toll-free)
www.niams.nih.gov

This division of the NIH deals with arthritis and other diseases of the musculoskeletal system. Its website includes a variety of informational resources about these conditions.

Harvard Medical School reports

The following Special Health Reports and Online Guides from Harvard Medical School delve into greater detail on various topics mentioned in this report. You can order them by going to www.health.harvard.edu or calling 877-649-9457 (toll-free).

Cardio Exercise: 7 workouts to boost energy, fight disease, and help you live longer

Controlling Your Allergies: How to gain the upper hand over asthma, hay fever, food allergies, and other allergic conditions

Core Exercises: 6 workouts to tighten your abs, strengthen your back, and improve your balance

The Harvard Medical School 6-Week Plan for Healthy Eating

Improving Memory: Understanding age-related memory loss

Improving Sleep: A guide to a good night's rest

Inflammatory Skin Conditions: Eczema, seborrheic dermatitis, and psoriasis

Living Well with Diabetes: Smart strategies for controlling your blood sugar

Lose Weight and Keep It Off: Smart approaches to achieving and maintaining a healthy weight

Quit Smoking for Good

Rheumatoid Arthritis: How to protect your joints, reduce pain, and improve mobility

Simple Changes, Big Rewards: A practical, easy guide for healthy, happy living

Stress Management: Enhance your well-being by reducing stress and building resilience

Ulcerative Colitis and Crohn's Disease: Treating inflammatory bowel disease

Walking for Health: Why this simple activity could be your best health insurance